CHRONIC PAIN

CHRONIC PAIN

FINDING HOPE IN THE MIDST OF SUFFERING

ROB PRINCE

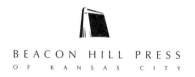

BEACON HILL PRESS
OF KANSAS CITY

10 9 8 7 6 5 4 3 2 1

DEDICATION

To Karla: When she said, "In sickness and in health," she meant it. She has kept her promises, and I love her for it!

To Alex and Ben: When they say, "Dad," those boys (now men) still make my day.

CONTENTS

ACKNOWLEDGMENTS

I am thankful for my family (both my immediate and extended versions). They have not only loved me and encouraged me but, as you will see, given me a great resource of stories for this book and countless sermons.

I am thankful for the great churches I have served in Alanson, Bad Axe (yes, there is a town called Bad Axe), Metropolitan, Richfield, Flint Central, (all in Michigan), and Kansas City (Central Church). They have been filled with God-following, pastor-loving, wonderfully kind people. The best thing I could say about them is that when my son Ben sensed a call into vocational ministry and I was questioning that decision, I asked him, "What will you do if you pastor a mean church with mean people?" Ben, in absolute astonishment, asked, "Are there churches like that?" He has only known churches filled with godly Christ followers who have loved him and the rest of our family. Thank you!

I am thankful for my many health providers. I'm sure there are bad doctors out there (somebody had to finish at the bottom of their graduating class), but mine have all been great!

I am also grateful to Bonnie Perry and the people of the Nazarene Publishing House who took their one-time sanitation engineer (janitor) and helped fulfill my call to not only preach the good news of Jesus Christ but also write of God and his great love.

And most importantly, I am forever grateful for the Mighty Healer, the Great I AM, our glorious heavenly Father!

INTRODUCTION

Pain is zero fun. The pain I've dealt with comes in the form of migraines. They are rotten, horrible, awful, and can ruin the best of plans. Throughout this book, I will discuss my journey of chronic pain, which for me means headaches. Though you may be suffering from a different type of chronic pain, I hope you can learn from my story.

I am not a doctor or the son of a doctor (as you can probably tell from the usage of my previously mentioned nonmedical lingo to describe migraines and headaches). Although as I am typing these words I am wearing a Harvard Medical School hoodie that I bought at my neighbor's garage sale—so maybe I am secretly desiring to be a doctor. Weird. My hoodie notwithstanding, this book is not intended to address medical issues as they relate to pain. Call a doctor if you are experiencing pain. The intention of this book is not to give a medical history of migraines or any kind of diagnosis as it relates to pain troubles. I may be a member of the clergy, but I am a layman when it comes to medical issues. When describing my journey, I use the terms *headache* and *migraine* interchangeably because in my mind they are both a pain and equally disrupt life. My true goal is to address the spiritual issues and questions that arise from battling chronic pain and offer the hope found in Jesus Christ to those who are suffering from this ailment.

I am a pastor—a pastor with chronic pain. (See the chapter that deals with this unique challenge.) Having lived most of my life battling migraines, surviving a subarachnoid hemorrhage, and constantly dealing with issues related to headaches, I am acutely aware that not all headache relief comes from a bottle of pills or the various treatments available. The spiritual aspect of pain relief is what this book addresses.

As such, before you read another word, please let me offer this disclaimer. This book is not. . .

1. A "here's how I got rid of my pain in five easy steps and you can do it too" book
2. An "if you have faith and pray enough, then you will be pain-free in a week" book or
3. A "send me twenty-five dollars and I will pray for you and your pain will be gone" book

This book is more of an "I know what you are going through and God is still God even when you experience excruciating pain" book. It's more of a travel guide of a fellow chronic pain sufferer. It is written by one of the millions of Americans who have spent enough nights in a dark room, trying to hear nothing but silence, wondering why the pain medicine is not working at all, and praying that the pain would leave.

So if you are also one of the millions who suffer from chronic pain or if you live with one or if you are friends with one, my hope is that this book will help and that those battling chronic pain will come to see God at work as I have in my journey.

My prayer is that chronic pain sufferers will hear what Jeremiah heard. The Lord spoke to the prophet with these words: "I am the LORD, the God of all mankind. Is anything too hard for me?" (Jeremiah 32:27). Those are helpful words when one realizes the obvious answer to God's rhetorical question is, "Of course not." Of course, nothing is too hard for the God of all mankind—including pain that makes all logical thought seem next to impossible. So why should I worry? God is in control. Nothing is too hard for him. I know that I can trust him.

On December 20, 2007, I suffered a subarachnoid hemorrhage (more on that later). Many die from such a condition, but God chose to touch me in a powerful way. I was back preaching in three weeks and back to my regular schedule in six weeks. Still, he has not chosen to eliminate all headaches from my life. In fact, migraines are a constant reminder of my frailty. Please know the thesis of this book is that through every pain I can testify that God is good, that his love endures forever, and that *nothing* is too hard for him.

If you are a fellow chronic pain sufferer, my prayer is that you will see God's powerful and healing touch upon your life. Should God heal you today or tomorrow or not until heaven, I pray that you will experience his presence and glory throughout the journey. I hope this book will aid in that discovery.

1 CHRONIC PAIN STINKS
(EXCUSE THE MEDICAL LINGO)

But God is like a sweet aroma for the pain sufferer.

If you are one of my fellow Americans that struggle with chronic pain, then you already know that it stinks. There's not a silver lining on the cloud. It doesn't matter if you're a "cup is half empty" or "cup is half full" type of person. It doesn't matter if you are a positive-thinking optimist or if you have a black cloud over your head, always negative Nellie. Even if your team wins the Super Bowl, your rich uncle from Hoboken puts you in his will, and the weatherman says the day is perfect, chronic pain still stinks.

Even with the Botox injections that I receive every three months (thirty to forty shots in my melon), I still have three or four headaches a week. Sometimes more. Occasionally they are the massive variety. By that I mean sitting-in-a-dark-room-with-no-noise-and-occasionally-nauseated massive variety. When my head is pounding, it does not matter how the Detroit Lions (my team of choice) have fared, how much cash is sitting in my bank account, or how sunny the day is—chronic pain stinks.

PAIN IS NOT THE ONLY BATTLE

There are times when all I can do is cover my head and try to eliminate any message to my brain—if I can't see anything, hear anything, smell anything, or touch anything, then maybe the migraine will be manageable. It will only be like a drum and bugle corps (not the whole marching band) is stepping through my cranium. It's difficult to describe the experience. At their worst, think of a constant Slurpee brain freeze: intense pain without the sugary goodness of a Slurpee. Most generally, my headaches are a constant present throbbing pain that is exacerbated by noise, light, and smells.

It's tough to sleep when pain is raging.

It's difficult to think when an intense pain is uncontrolled.

My doctors have put me on a strict diet in an attempt to eliminate different food triggers.

My pharmacists and I are on a first-name basis.

Pain has disrupted nearly every aspect of my life.
Still, sufferers know that the pain is not the only battle.
Sometimes the "cure" is as bad as the pain. I have tried several different daily medications with varied amounts of success. None of the medications have provided a miracle cure, and all of them had serious side effects.
One medication caused several memory lapses. Memory lapses and preaching sermons are not a good combination. I have been in the middle of a sermon and forgotten where I was heading with a point, or more frequently I have not been able to pull out the right word for the point I was making. I forgot names of people—prior to the medication, remem-

bering names was one of my strong suits. The memory gaps were more than a little frustrating.

I knew that the memory lapses were bad when I was picking up a new set of prescription glasses from the optical department at Wal-Mart. Since I was in the store, my wife, Karla, asked me to also pick up some chicken for dinner. If you are keeping score at home, I had two tasks: get my eyeglasses from the optical department and purchase some chicken. Simple, right?

I went to the optical department first, gave my receipt indicating that I had paid for my glasses to the worker, and then went to get my chicken. While waiting in the checkout line with my lone item, I received a call on my cell phone from the optical department. They informed me that I forgot my glasses in the department. How strange. I had one task in the optical department: to pick up my eyeglasses. I had already paid for them. All I had to do was pick up the glasses. That's it—just grab them. How could I not do the only task I had? I had no idea how that could take place. So I thanked the optical department worker and assured him I would pick up my glasses after I paid for my chicken.

On my way out of the store, I grabbed my glasses and proceeded to my car, at which time I discovered that I left the chicken (the only other item I was purchasing, remember) at the checkout. How does one forget his chicken when he was only buying chicken? I only had two tasks and I forgot to grab either purchase. Something had to change. The medications (that were not eliminating my headaches anyway) were not worth the memory hassles. My doctor tried another one. It wasn't much better. My fingers and toes constantly felt like they were asleep. We tried still another one. It tended to aid in weight gain and made my mouth feel dry all the time. We tried some more. Again, there were plenty of side effects and little relief. I'm trying another new one right now. Will it work? I hope so, but I'm not holding my breath.

Botox has helped me somewhat—it has eliminated the strength and duration of my headaches, but it has not eliminated them. More on that experience later.

All of this to say, those are just a few of the annoying side stories of a life scrambled by chronic pain. There are many more that I could share.

Bottom line: chronic pain stinks. From the obvious pain, to the drain on the family, to medication hang-ups, to the dietary restrictions, to the sleep disturbances, it all adds up to a rather stinky situation.

Do others deal with more difficulties? Obviously, yes. Does that bring comfort when traveling through a rough pain journey? Not really.

LAZARUS'S STINKING SITUATION

There is only one story in the Bible where God's Holy Word says that a particular person's life stinks. It's an amazing story of God's miraculous working in a person's life. With a simple word, Jesus transformed four-day, stinking-dead Lazarus into a living, breathing, alive Lazarus. In my estimation it is the most remarkable of all the miraculous deeds Jesus performed.

During most of my growing up years, we didn't have children's church. Everyone from toddlers on up went to "big people's" church. My parents were in the sit-still-and-be-quiet camp and didn't believe in bringing crayons and coloring books to occupy my time in church. So this fidgeting, couldn't-sit-still-if-my-life-depended-on-it kid had to (very unsuccessfully on most Sundays) sit still in the very hard pews at the little church we attended.

One way (I should not admit this) that I tried to pass time was playing the "nasty Bible verse game." Ever play it? A long-winded preacher and threats of "not sparing the rod" were enough incentive to play the game. The object of the "nasty Bible verse game" was to find the grossest, weirdest, or funniest Bible verse that I could locate. It's a rather juvenile game. But the game fulfilled its purpose in keeping me quiet in church and keeping my nose in the Bible. The story of Lazarus includes one of the funny verses in the Bible. At least, to my adolescent mind, I considered it funny.

As you remember the story, when Jesus finally, oh so finally, arrived on the scene, Lazarus had been in the grave for four days. Jesus insisted on going to the cemetery. Not only did he insist on going to the graveyard, but he also insisted on seeing the body and having the rock that was blocking the entrance of the tomb removed.

Martha, the sister of Lazarus, thought that was a really bad idea. Here's how John told it:

Jesus, once more deeply moved, came to the tomb. It was a cave with a stone laid across the entrance. "Take away the stone," he said. "But, Lord," said Martha, the sister of the dead man, "by this time there is a bad odor, for he has been there four days." (John 11:38-39)

The last phrase is the part of the verse that always amused me. That is the one spot where God's Holy Word points out that "there is a bad odor" in that tomb. To my juvenile mind that verse was the stuff of great heavenly humor. In fact, I like even better the way the King James Version reads. It says: "Lord, by this time he stinketh."

My older sisters would frequently tattle when I happened to "stinketh" too. I could relate to old Lazarus when his sister ratted him out for his nasal-offending ways. Of course, I never had as good of an excuse as Lazarus for my offensive odor.

Still, I could relate as a boy to Lazarus, and in many ways on my pain journey I still can relate, maybe more so.

The smelly days of a boy who didn't like to take a bath are behind me (mostly). Still, I understand that life can sometimes stink.

WHEN LIFE STINKS

Sometimes life stinks—not because of sin (although we will address this issue as it relates to pain in another chapter)—sometimes life stinks because of poor choices. (We will address that later too.) Sometimes life stinks because of other people's poor decisions. And sometimes life just stinks—not because of any action of our own or anyone else.

Sometimes life just stinks.

I don't know if you've thought about this fact, but as far as we know, Lazarus did nothing to get himself into his "smelly condition." He wasn't at fault. He got sick. He died. Maybe it was a heart attack; maybe it was kidney trouble; maybe it was a brain hemorrhage. He got sick, and he died. It was not his fault. No one was to blame. Four days later, when Jesus showed up, Lazarus stunk.

Like my brain hemorrhage, sometimes life just happens. And it stinks.

I've known people who, through no fault of their own, have found themselves in some pretty stinky situations. June (not her real name) was such a person. June was completely messed up. She could not relate to people. Every relationship in her life was a total wreck—in her marriage, with her kids, and with every other acquaintance, she seemed to be in constant conflict.

People would try to get close to June, but she would always get mad. She had a knack of sabotaging even the most wonderful friendships and most helpful people in her life.

She would find a way to end those relationships that she desperately needed.

People were afraid of saying the wrong thing around June. She would frequently take what others said the wrong way. On one occasion, June called me quite upset because of a thank-you note she received. A thank-you note! She simply could not relate to people. I remember thinking, "What happened to June that caused her to be so volatile?"

And then I met June's mother. I had heard rumors about this woman. None of the stories were good. She was always described in very unflattering terms by those who had encountered her. I would learn that all the descriptions of this lady were wrong. They weren't severe enough.

But June's mom was in the hospital, and June asked if I would visit her. That's what pastors do. We visit and pray for sick people in hospitals. So I went.

Usually people are nice when a preacher shows up at the hospital. Most people figure they could use all the prayer they can get when they are in a hospital and when a preacher shows up, they are most generally on their best behavior. Not this lady. June's mom was angry, mean, and very strange. It was one of the most bizarre hospital visits I have ever made. It wasn't medication or pain that put this lady in her state of mind. She was completely unstable. Some would say evil. I seriously doubt that I helped her mom all that much by my visit, but it sure helped me to understand why June was the way she was.

I thought, "If that's the way her mom is to a complete stranger who is simply trying to be nice, and if that's who was June's primary caregiver, then it's no wonder June doesn't know how to relate to people. It's no wonder she doesn't know how to hold a pleasant conversation. It's no wonder she doesn't even know how to receive a compliment. If that was her role model, June's life growing up had to stink!"

Sometimes people's lives stink. Through no fault of their own, their life just stinks. Because of abuse or circumstances out of their control or sickness or just the junk of life, they might find themselves looking around and saying, "What did I do to deserve this? My life really stinks!"

If you are a chronic pain sufferer, then you've probably thought that too. "I didn't ask for this. I don't want this. This pain feels like it is killing me. Life stinks."

CHOOSING STINK

Of course, some people are responsible for the stink that they are in. Their choices, their decisions, their behaviors, their attitudes have led them to their stink. That happens too.

I had a friend who worked at a pig farm. It was a really big pig farm. He was proud of his pigs and wanted me to see the whole operation. The day we decided for me to see his farm, I had other things going too, most notably a lunch date planned with my wife, Karla. Still, I had never visited a pig farm and thought this was a wonderful opportunity to see my bacon before it got to my plate.

When I arrived, my friend had coveralls for me to wear over the top of my clothes. He told me I needed to wear the coveralls or I would smell like pig when we were through. Have you ever smelled pig smell before? Without trying to be offensive to Porky or Arnold, there are a lot of bad smells in the world, and pig smell is one of them. I didn't need to put on coveralls to keep the pig smell off of me; I needed to wear a yellow, emergency hazmat suit that a nuclear disaster response team wears. There was no way I was going to visit all the barns and piggies without leaving with some pig smell on me—coveralls or no coveralls.

Still, I went ahead and saw all the little piggies and the whole piggy operation. Even though I knew that I was to meet Karla (and her near superhuman sense of smell) afterward, and I knew those coveralls probably weren't stopping the stink of the pig barns and operation from infiltrating onto my clothes, I continued on. The piggies were cute.

I think during my little tour of the operation, I had grown accustomed to the smell and didn't realize just how overwhelmed with pig stink my clothes had become. As soon as I left my friend's pig farm, I went to see Karla, and no sooner had I walked into her office (she may have smelled me driving down the highway—I'm telling you, she is a superhero when it comes to smells) when she said, "Where in the world have you been? Ooh! You stink." Just in case you are wondering, you never want the first words out of your wife's mouth upon greeting you to be, "Ooh, you stink." That's never a good thing.

No one twisted my arm to go into the pig barn. I didn't have to go. I chose to go in. I wanted to go. I knew it would make me stink. Still I went in. It was my decision.

Sometimes it is our decisions that lead to a stinky life. Usually those choices lead to much more serious consequences than a wife's turning up her nose at a smelly husband. There are some choices that we make that contribute to chronic pain, and eliminating those triggers will help alleviate some of our troubles. In a later chapter we will discuss doing all that you can to help eliminate or avoid some of the triggers for pain. Not all pain is random and coincidental. Some pain is the result of the choices we have made.

JESUS IS THE WAY THROUGH
THE STINKING TIMES OF LIFE

Here is what you need to take away from this chapter: whether you find yourself in a stinky situation of your own doing or simply because of the way life is, Jesus is the way through your stinky situation. Notice I didn't use the word *out* but rather *through*. Will Jesus heal you? Maybe. But whether you are the recipient of a huge pain-busting miracle or whether you carry it with you to the pearly gates, Jesus will see you through!

I think my favorite sequence of verses (I've moved beyond thinking that "he stinketh" is the best part of the story) in this passage about Lazarus is what happened next:

Then Jesus said, "Did I not tell you that if you believe, you will see the glory of God?" So they took away the stone. Then Jesus looked up and said, "Father, I thank you that you have heard me. I knew that you always hear me, but I said this for the benefit of the people standing here, that they may believe that you sent me." When he had said this, Jesus called in a loud voice, "Lazarus, come out!" The dead man came out. (John 11:40-44)

I love that last phrase because four-day-dead men don't "come out" of anything. Four-day-dead men don't move. Four-day-dead men don't roll over. Four-day-dead people don't yawn, sneeze, or blink. Four-day-dead men don't even twitch a little bit. You know what four-day-dead people do? They stay put. Four-day-dead men stay exactly where the mortician placed them. But not in this case! The dead man came out!

How did he come out? He was still wrapped up in the burial clothes and still stinky, no doubt. Looking like a PG-rated horror movie, the mummy-like Lazarus walked out of the tomb.

John doesn't tell us everything that happens next. He just moves on with the story of Jesus. (It is the story of Jesus, after all, and not the story of Lazarus.) He tells us that Lazarus took off the graveclothes (with a little help from some folks). But then he probably went and took a bath (trying to wash off the four-day-dead stink) and got cleaned up the best he could. Maybe he splashed on some New Spice. (Could there really be Old Spice in the first century? I don't think so.) But I imagine he did whatever he could to get rid of the four-day-dead stink. Jesus raised him from the dead, but the stink of death was still on him.

WHEN THE STINK LINGERS

I point that out because while Lazarus had been raised from the dead, there were still a few tasks he needed to accomplish before the stink of death was gone. He had to get out of the mummy clothes and get cleaned up. For many of us, that's a problem. We like things cleaned up quickly. We don't like thinking that Lazarus still had a little stink on him as he came out of the tomb.

We love quick-change stories like that of a NASCAR pit crew. We like stories like my dad's life story. Christians love to hear my dad's story. By his admission, my dad was a drunk, found Jesus, and never ever, ever had another drink again. He found Jesus, and "Boom!" No more alcohol! His conversion was before the popularity of twelve-step programs, Celebrate Recovery groups, or anything else. He just accepted Jesus, and that was it. No more alcoholism. He never fell off the wagon in his fifty years of being a Christian. He was completely and totally changed. His was a great story.

But not everybody's story is like his. It's not always that clean-cut. For a lot of folks, it's two steps forward, one step back, three steps forward, two steps back. This is especially true in dealing with chronic pain.

I've discovered on this pain journey that there has not been a "boom! all of my headaches are instantly gone and life is instantly good" moment. There has been relief in stages. But sometimes it's two steps forward, as I'm doing well for a week or two, and it's a step (or sometimes two or three steps) back as new medications, diet, and treatments are tried with varying degrees of success.

My point is that sometimes when we begin to exit our "tomb" we still might have a little stink to us. Could Jesus instantly and forever change us in a "boom! all is better" type of moment? Absolutely. It just hasn't happened that way for me. Not yet.

We are really good at rejoicing in the powerful, radical transformations like my dad's. We say, "Yippee! Look at that guy! He went from a drunk to a board member. Wow! He never fell off the wagon! He did great!" But with those people that struggle, we haven't always been so quick to come alongside them. And that's too bad. Because when life stinks, that's when folks need a friend by their side to hold on to them and whisper in their ear, "Keep on going! Jesus is with you! You can make it!"

Rather than pretending that the church is for people whose lives are perfect and that everybody in church is perfect in every way, maybe we should admit that the church is full of people who are imperfect and quite frankly have a little bit of a stink to them.

Can I say it that way?

Many people who know my struggle with chronic pain will ask, "How are your headaches?" They would love to hear and I would love to tell them, "Man, they are gone. Completely gone. God has completely made me well!" But it hasn't been that way. Sometimes they are a little better. Sometimes they are a little worse. So usually, I just say, "Oh, they are doing about the same. But that's okay. God is helping me."

This pain journey is a stinky one. There are times when I paste a smile on my face and go to church or around town and act like everything is terrific: I pretend there are no troubles and act like there is no stink when inside I know the truth—it's been a rough day, my head is pounding, and I have a sermon to preach.

The "beauty" of headaches is that you mostly look the same with one as you look without one. It's not like when you have a broken bone and everyone can see the cast. One looks about the same with a headache as he or she looks without one. Maybe that's not so beautiful after all. Maybe that's part of the problem.

Our churches are filled with people who are dealing with stinky issues. Mine happens to be headaches and migraines. Often you might not be able to tell that people have troubles, but they do. People have issues, and all of us need to be reminded (again and again sometimes) that even when life stinks, Jesus is there and he will help us navigate through the stink.

Did you read that?

Jesus is the way *through* our messy, stinky situations. Hearing Jesus' voice in the midst of the stink is the way through! And sometimes—let me restate that—often he provides the voices of fellow stink bearers, fellow Christians who are battling their own stinky situations to offer just the right soothing, kind, perfect word and the prayer we need for that moment.

HELP FROM FELLOW STINK BEARERS

My help has often come not from fellow pain sufferers but from people who know a thing or two about suffering.

I was in the midst of a particularly "migrainey" couple of weeks. I'm not exactly sure why—maybe it was the spring weather, allergies, my diet, my last round of Botox wearing off, or all of the above contributing to a daily pain in my noggin. All to say, I was looking forward to my quarterly Botox injections that particular day. Normally, a sane person would not be excited to receive thirty to forty shots in the melon, but truth be told, I was ready.

As a matter of full disclosure, let me also admit that I may be getting less tolerant in my old age, because that particular week's injections left me feeling more of a pincushion than normal. I always close my eyes and count down the number of injections left. I try to pray or think happy thoughts or make conversation with the doctor and his assistant while they are poking my dome again and again. But that particular week I just felt cranky.

As another matter of full disclosure, I was probably feeling a little sorry for myself on that Tuesday morning as I put my pincushion-like head into my car and drove out of my neurologist's parking lot to visit a parishioner at a local hospital. I had already determined that following the shots, I would visit my friend Logan Clark who had surgery the week prior. Here's the deal—I just wasn't ready to go on a hospital visit. I wasn't ready to be "Pastor Rob." I was more in a mode to feel sorry for myself, hop in bed, and not see anyone all day. But a promise is a promise, and I went to the hospital. I was cranky, moody, and grumpy, but I went.

Logan is a great young man who was involved in a horrific car accident that left him paralyzed from the waist down. Given a similar diagnosis, many young people have become bitter, enraged, or flat-out obnoxious. Not Logan. During his recovery, he learned to play the piano and now is a very accomplished player. He is also a gifted artist. He is talented, funny, smart, and a big baseball fan. He went to a Christian college close to home and was moving on with his life following the accident.

Prior to his most recent hospital stay, Logan had decided that a school in Nashville had a better program for him, so in a courageous manner, he packed up his belongings and went off on a new scholastic adventure several hundred miles from home. While in school in Nashville, Logan developed a sore. For more than a year, doctors tried practically everything to help the healing process, but nothing worked. He came to the point where he had to drop out of school. He moved back home as his doctors examined, researched, consulted, and finally prepared for surgery. Without being overly graphic, the medical staff at the hospital took a chunk of muscle and skin from his leg and inserted it into the once-infected area. Besides having many more stitches than my grandma's cross-stitch "artwork," Logan was going to have to lie flat on his back for the next couple of months. If you haven't added up all of those details, let me say that for most adults (young or old), any one of those issues would have been the source of much anger and resentment. But not for Logan.

When I got to the hospital, Logan and his mom were in the room. But they weren't having a pity party. There was no "weeping and gnashing of teeth." Far from it. Instead we talked about the future, how God was working in Logan's life, and how he and his dad were planning on going to the summer's Major League Baseball All-Star Game that was to be played in Kansas City.

I thanked Logan for participating in our Easter service. On Easter Sunday, we had a "cardboard testimony" service. Several churches have done this. Many people from the congregation (Logan was one of them) shared on a piece of cardboard what God had done in their lives. On one side of the cardboard, the participants wrote of a tragedy, sin, or problems that had been in their lives, and on the flip side, they shared the hope that they now have in Christ and what Jesus has done in response to their situation. Logan's cardboard testimony read:

Side One: Paralyzed in a head-on collision at sixteen.

Flip Side: Jesus has walked for me ever since!

I cried like a baby when he rolled to the center of the sanctuary in his wheelchair and held up his sign.

And it's true. Logan continues to walk with Jesus. Jesus has helped, empowered, and given him an inner strength that few people his age (or any age) display. Not only that, it's obvious through his attitude and actions that God is not done with Logan.

In fact, on that particular visit to the hospital, God used Logan to speak to me. My intention was to go to the hospital to "cheer him up." (Isn't that why pastors go to hospitals? Aren't we supposed to offer cheer and prayers on behalf of the sick?) But that week, the roles were reversed.

Remember, I was at the hospital following my Botox treatment of thirty to forty shots in my head. I was feeling a little sorry for myself. Then through Logan and his mom, God reminded me that we do not always control our circumstances. Rather, he is still in control. Adversity comes into everyone's life to some degree or another, but the character of the person is determined by how he or she handles that adversity.

On that particular day I was not handling my "light and momentary troubles" (to quote the apostle Paul) very well. Logan showed me that with Jesus, I'll make it.

Most of us will not have to deal with the life circumstances that Logan confronts every single day, but I hope we can discover the strength, grace, and faith that will allow us to face any adversity that might come our way. It's a matter of focusing on Jesus rather than the stinking situation we find ourselves in.

NO MORE COLOGNE SHOWERS

When I was a college student, following a workout and before heading to dinner, we would take a "cologne shower." A "cologne shower" was splashing on cologne instead of taking a shower before heading to the cafeteria for lunch or dinner. Hunger outweighed hygiene (maybe my sisters were right about the "He stinketh" tattles), so we'd splash on a little cologne and hope it would cover up the stink of a sweaty workout. (No need to wonder why I didn't have many dates in college.)

I think church folks are guilty of the same mind-set of a "cologne shower." Too often, trying to hide the stink rather than dealing with it has been our method. But the true church operates best when it is less like a sterile, perfectly clean, antiseptic-smelling museum and more like a stinky, smelly emergency room. The church is at its best when hurting, troubled, messed-up people feel welcome and deeply loved. The church is at its best when it allows people to share their stinky situations in a spirit of love and assistance. The church is at its best when it operates under Jesus' mandate to be "full of grace and truth."

Here's what I know about Jesus. He loves smelly people.

Martha said to him, "Jesus, you can't roll that rock away. Lazarus stinks!"

And what you will *not* read in the next verse is Jesus saying something like, "Oh, wow, you're right, Martha. I forgot about that. I had better stay away. Because, whew . . . I hate smelly people!" Of course not! He said, "Roll the rock away!" In a loud voice he yelled, "Lazarus, come out."

Jesus was not offended by Lazarus' condition, and he is not offended by you!

He loves you!

The stinky situation you might find yourself in—whether you are there because of your own choices or simply because sometimes life stinks—doesn't cause Jesus to turn his head and run from you. In fact, it is just the opposite.

He comes to you.

He stands outside of your painful, heart-wrenching place or that migraine full of desperation, and he calls to you. He knows your name and says, "Come out. I'm here. You can trust me. I will see you through the stinkiest of times."

The following chapters will address living with the reality that while I have not been healed, Jesus is still with me. More specifically, I will tell of my case of following Jesus with chronic pain. When faced with the prospect of following Jesus with some other debilitating disease, maybe one could conclude that migraines aren't as bad. Maybe that's true. I've never had some other debilitating disease. Here's what I know: chronic pain stinks, and Jesus can help even when the headaches keep coming back week after week. So if you or someone you love has had to deal with pain day after day; if you prayed for God to end the pain day after day; and if for whatever reason God hasn't miraculously answered that prayer yet, then read on!

2 | MY CHRONIC PAIN
DEALING WITH MIGRAINES

I've always had headaches. As a boy, migraines would figuratively send me through the roof and literally send me home from school. In those days, I would only begin to find relief after I had lost my lunch. In junior high school, my doctor had placed me on a medication that was so strong that one day I fell asleep while walking from one class to another. I woke up, leaning against a wall with no one in the hallway except me. Had this happened at the Christian college I attended a few years later, I might have been tempted to think that the rapture had occurred and I had been left behind. No such worries overcame me in the corridors of Radcliff Junior High School. I was pretty confident that I would not be alone in my school had the "last trumpet sounded."

The headaches continued into college and seminary. They have been a constant component of my life as a pastor. As much as I wanted to, I couldn't blame my headaches on nasty parishioners, board members, or potlucks gone bad. I battled migraines long before I dealt with any such issues in a pastoral way.

From time to time, a new doctor would prescribe a new remedy. But nothing seemed to work much. My over-the-counter medicine of choice was ibuprofen, of which I took a lot. Later I learned that probably wasn't the best decision. I would get a headache and pop three or four tablets. I even had doctors prescribe 800-milligram tablets so I could get a bigger bang for my buck. It brought some relief, but not a lot. The headaches continued. Usually one headache was followed by an even stronger headache. The cycle was repeated over and over again. Later I learned about "rebound headaches" where the continued use of drugs like ibuprofen was actually contributing to (not eliminating) my life with headaches.

Then, in 2007, as I was experiencing a busy five-days-before-Christmas morning (we all know it's Santa's busy season, but it's also a tad busy for preachers too), my headache went to a new level.

That year had been particularly stressful. There was a lot going on at the church besides the normal Christmastime craziness. It was more than the "I hope we don't run out of candles on Christmas Eve" hassles, in other words. There were church staff issues swirling; the economy was not great and I feared a major financial crisis looming; and at that exact moment, I was reading an email from an irate parent who believed our youth pastor was the spawn of Satan. (Incidentally, I've met his parents and they happen to be very nice people not even remotely close to the devil.) Anyway, as I was reading the riveting email and got somewhere between "Satan" and "spawn," I instantly felt like I had been smashed in the head with a Louisville Slugger.

I knew that it was not normal to have the immediate sensation that I was being cracked in the noggin with a baseball bat. I am not a doctor, but I quickly surmised that I was either having a stroke or a brain aneurism. I took two ibuprofen tablets (of course) that were sitting on my desk—as if ibuprofen were going to be the remedy for a stroke. (I went to seminary, not medical school.) I then attempted to walk to my assistant's desk for help but didn't make it quite that far and instead fell into a chair in between those two points. Thankfully, Pam heard my distress and quickly got me to the hospital.

I was diagnosed with a subarachnoid hemorrhage. If you also went to seminary or some other nonmedical school, let me tell you that's not a good thing. I have learned that 50 percent of the people who have a subarachnoid hemorrhage die, and many times those who survive have major complications. Ten percent of those who have subarachnoid hemorrhages don't even make it to the hospital alive.

After arriving at a second hospital (the first was convinced I needed surgery that they would not do), the bleeding in my brain stopped on its own. No surgery was needed, but I was far from back to normal.

I was a tad out of my mind during those first thirty-six hours following the hemorrhage. Among other things (unbeknownst to me), my secret desire to be Latino came out as I asked the nurse to call me "Roberto." I know this because once I came to my senses my nurse timidly asked, "Do you ever have people call you Roberto?" I thought that was such a bizarre question. "No," I emphatically assured her. "Well, you wanted me to call you Roberto," she said, laughing. Some of the folks at my church still refer to me as "Roberto." (I probably should not have shared that story with them.) I called my assistant sometime during the night and sang into her voice mail a little ditty about how I wasn't going to be at work the next day and how I wasn't dead yet. (Chris Tomlin has no worries from me in any songwriting competition.) My boys had fun at my expense asking me every few minutes the time of day. I would always be shocked by the lateness of the hour. I left several messages on my mom's answering machine informing her of my condition and telling her not to worry. Ironically, receiving the same message over and over again caused her to worry a lot.

My wife, Karla, thought all of this was a little amusing as well. Until it dawned on her it was not any medicine that was making me loopy—it was my messed-up brain making me loopy. Upon this epiphany, she spoke to the nurse to see if this condition would be permanent, to which the nurse replied, "That's what we are waiting to see." I think that's when Karla really began praying for me.

After a day or so, I regained my faculties, the nurse still chuckled that I wanted her to call me Roberto, and all was mostly well. I did not have any major complications that most survivors battle. After a week in the hospital, I was released. It was an answer to many prayers. Three weeks later I was back in the pulpit. Six weeks later I was back to my full schedule. All have said, "It was quite remarkable."

But I still have headaches—only now worse than ever.

It was so bad that in the summer of 2010, I had a migraine that began the end of April and lasted until the end of August. I remember walking through the woods in Branson, Missouri, while on a pastors' retreat and being overcome with a massive migraine. It wasn't a brain hemorrhage headache, but it was close. It wouldn't stop. It stayed with me day after day, week after week. That's a doozy of a headache.

I would go to church and work most of the day, then come home and go straight to bed. I would turn off all the lights, try to eliminate all sound, and pray that the next day would be better than that day. Rarely was it better.

My neurologist tried a number of remedies. Nothing worked. He tried new medicines, diet, and an IV therapy where twice a week I would be hooked up to a concoction of medicines meant to block the headache. Eventually, I received quarterly Botox injections.

Botox (the brand name for onabotulinum toxin type A) is a prescription medicine that is injected into the muscles to prevent headaches in adults with chronic migraines. A chronic migraine sufferer typically has more than fifteen headaches a month lasting for more than four hours a day. Botox works in blocking the chemical changes on the nerve endings that cause headaches. It stops the pained nerve ending from sending a message to the brain that there is something painful happening. Think of Botox as the offensive linemen trying to keep the defensive players from sacking your quarterback (aka your brain). I receive Botox shots in the forehead, side and back of the head, and in the back of my neck.

Botox doesn't "cure" migraines, but it helps in controlling them. One side effect of its use is that I can't raise my eyebrows. I have told my sons that they can still shock me; I just won't look shocked by their behavior. My eyebrows just won't go up. I've tried and tried, and those brows will not rise. I have also experienced head drop with Botox. That is, at times at the end of the day, my head feels extra heavy. I feel like I need to be like *The Thinker* sculpture, with my chin resting on my fist. Thankfully, the head-drop issues only last for a week or two.

Enduring Botox injections is not particularly enjoyable. Having your dome turned into a human pincushion is not a barrel of laughs. For me, I receive thirty to forty shots in my head and neck every three months. Usually, I go into my doctor's office, close my eyes, and open them only when the injections are done. I have now received several treatments, and I have yet to see a needle. If you are tallying at home, that's more than five hundred shots, and I have yet to see a needle. It's better that way.

I've had plenty of ladies jokingly ask if I had some extra Botox to help them eliminate a wrinkle or two. Botox doesn't really help my wrinkles. I was worried after the first treatment that I would come out looking like Joan Rivers, but the only wrinkly area that is affected is my forehead. I have a pretty smooth forehead these days.

Obviously, headache reduction, not wrinkle removal, is my goal. So far it has worked remarkably well in reducing the intensity and frequency of my headaches. Botox and I have become friends. Being a pincushion for forty-five minutes is nothing compared to enduring massive headaches for three months. So now my motto to my doctor (as sung by eighties rocker Pat Benatar) is: "Hit me with your best shot."

In case you ever would have surmised otherwise, I did not ask for this. I did not bring this on myself (although a case could be made that my stress level and mismanagement of said stress did aid in my "blowing a head gasket"). This was not my idea.

It's tough to go about life when your head is pounding like the University of Michigan Marching Band is marching through your cranium. It's tough to do much of anything when even the slightest noises sound like the *1812 Overture* is going off in your eardrum.

My day job is a pastor. As everyone knows, we only work one day a week (Ha!). There have been occasions when I preached two sermons in the morning, taught a Sunday school class in between the two services, and then preached once and occasionally twice on Sunday nights. (The people of my church really are not slave drivers. I signed up for the job.) Thanks to my headache "friend," I have on occasion had to preach with a boomer of a headache. Not an easy task. The bottles say not to take such strong medication while operating heavy machinery; it doesn't say anything about handling heavy scripture passages. So I press on and preach on.

Leading meetings (*Bam, bam, bam!*), visiting sick folks in the hospital and wondering if I should find an empty room with an extra bed (*Bam, bam, bam!*), and carrying on all the duties of shepherding a thriving congregation while the drum and bugle corps is marching and pounding in one's noggin is challenging, to say the least.

I've prayed. I've been anointed. I've claimed scripture, and all the rest. I've done everything short of placing my hand on the TV screen in the direction of a faith healer, and still the headache continues.

NOT A LOT OF SMILING IN THE STORM

To be clear, this book is not a "how to smile in the storm" kind of book.

There are those who think—whether a pastor or a faithful, Bible-believing follower of Christ—that smiling in the storm is the Christian thing to do. When I came upon my four-month-migraine tsunami, I discovered that even with Jesus in my boat I wasn't smiling too much. I wanted to smile, but I didn't feel much like smiling.

Of course, this illustration is taken from the story told in Luke 8. Here's how Luke told the story:

One day Jesus said to his disciples, "Let us go over to the other side of the lake." So they got into a boat and set out. As they sailed, he fell asleep. A squall came down on the lake, so that the boat was being swamped, and they were in great danger. The disciples went and woke him, saying, "Master, Master, we're going to drown!" He got up and rebuked the wind and the raging waters; the storm subsided, and all was calm. "Where is your faith?" he asked his disciples. In fear and amazement they asked one another, "Who is this? He commands even the winds and the water, and they obey him." (Verses 22-25) Did you read it carefully? Read it again. Notice anything about the disciples?

They began the story sailing, presumably smiling because everybody smiles when sailing, right? At least it seems that way in the Tommy Hilfiger commercials. Tommy always seems to be smiling. Wind in his face, water splashing, sun shining, no storms in sight. Everything is great.

But in Luke 8, as Jesus was napping on this brief sailing excursion, a storm came up. When the squall arose, the disciples weren't napping, and they presumably weren't smiling anymore either, because the Bible says they were in "great danger." (I've never seen anybody smile who was in great danger.) They may have been screaming, crying, or shaking in their sandals, but they were not smiling. They were afraid.

Gripped with fear, someone gets the task of waking up Jesus, as he is sleeping below deck. Upon this no doubt rude awakening from a fraidy-cat disciple, Jesus promptly rebuked the wind and the raging waters; the storm quit storming, and Jesus asked the disciples, "Where is your faith?"

Once again the disciples are fearful, only this time they are fearful because of the power and might displayed by Jesus, not because of the power and might of the storm. Luke wrote that they were amazed too.

Probably you and I would have been a bit amazed and a little fearful in that moment too. But do you notice anything missing in that whole account?

No one was smiling. Maybe Jesus was smiling—he did just perform a pretty cool miracle, after all. Although he was also just awakened from a nap—usually I'm not smiling when someone wakes me from a nap. So I'm not sure that even Jesus was smiling.

Luke 8:26 then moves on to another story. It does not say, "And Peter from henceforth had a big, goofy grin on his face." As far as I can tell, they were never smiling in the storm. They were fearful in the storm. Probably hollering. Maybe screaming, shaking, and nervous.

But they sure weren't smiling. They didn't need to be fearful, since Jesus was in the boat, but they were. In fact, they were fearful after the storm too, and Jesus was *still* in the boat. After the storm, the whole reason they were fearful is precisely *because* Jesus was in the boat. It dawned on the disciples that the One who had been napping below deck was more powerful than the storm that was raging on the deck. At that point they were really afraid. No smiling—just afraid.

SMILING IN THE BIBLE

The word *smile* is only found in one book out of the sixty-six books in your Bible, and you would never guess which one. In fact, if we were to play a guessing game in which book in the Bible you would find the word *smile*, it might be your last guess.

It's in the book of Job. Job! Just in case you haven't read ol' Job lately, it's not a book that's particularly known for its grins, giggles, and belly laughs. And to be perfectly honest, none of the three references in the book are of Job remembering a happy time, reminiscing about a good day, or "smiling in his storm."

Now, please understand—I am not advocating being grumpy in our storms either. Remember Paul's words to the Philippian church: "I have learned to be content whatever the circumstances" (Philippians 4:11). Being content means not being grumpy, but it says nothing about smiling or liking the storm that has consumed you.

All this to say, there are times when even our Christian friends would prefer that we paste a smile on our face during the storms of our life and act like everything is okay, when we know good and well that everything is not okay. They ask, "How are you doing?" The expected response is, "Good. Great. Never better." But the truth is, everything stinks. There is a reason we call it a storm. Like the boat the disciples were in, we are being swamped and feel like we are about to go down. Sure, Jesus is there. But that doesn't mean we are smiling, and it doesn't mean it's easy. And it doesn't mean we like what's happening.

There were plenty of times during the last few years as I've battled migraine after migraine when I have not felt like smiling. There have been more times than not, like the disciples in the boat, I would have been screaming, hollering, or crying out had those activities not contributed to my pounding head. So instead I would pray in quiet. No smiles—just a lot of frustration.

With Jesus in the boat, even when you are not smiling and when you are crying out, and you don't think it could get worse and then it does get worse, you can still depend on the Faithful One who is in the boat with you. Jesus is in my boat, and that fact makes this journey worth it. He has promised that I am not traveling through the storm alone. I have joy knowing that Jesus is alive and well and giving me strength, but that joy does not always equal smiles.

Jesus is with me in every headache, migraine, and Botox injection. Each time I preach with a booming headache (or when I preach without a headache), he has given me the strength and the words to proclaim his good news. Throughout this ordeal, Jesus has never left me. He doesn't leave me when I'm not smiling because of the storm. He doesn't leave when I get frustrated by the lack of answers or help from medications. He simply has promised to never leave me—smiles or no smiles. And he won't leave you!

3 ⦚ PAIN AND THE BIBLE
WHAT THE BIBLE SAYS ABOUT CHRONIC PAIN

The Bible lists many ills that plagued God's people. Peter's mother-in-law had a fever. Recall the woman with the bleeding disorder. Many people were blind, lame, or had contracted leprosy. Paul admits to having a "thorn in his side," just to name a few.

There is one story from the Bible that is particularly meaningful to me. If you were born blind, then you might find the healing of Blind Bartimaeus to be the most meaningful Bible story. If you were in a wheelchair or struggled with mobility, then maybe the stories of how Jesus healed those who couldn't walk would hold a special place in your heart. If you struggle with infertility, maybe the story of Samuel's mom, Hannah, or Abraham and Sarah would be the most meaningful miracle story. But if you had a subarachnoid brain hemorrhage, like me, then I think the story of God's working in 2 Kings 4 might be the most significant story. It's the only place that the Bible specifically tells us that someone had a headache (not counting Goliath—he had a little run-in with a stone to the noggin from David's slingshot—but that doesn't count).

Maybe there were other people in the Bible who had headaches like me—there are certainly others who dealt with chronic pain issues—but we aren't given details except in this one case.

In 2 Kings 4, we are told about a woman who was very kind to Elisha. She and her husband provided food and lodging for him. Elisha was so thankful for her kindness that he wanted to show the man and wife his appreciation. He discovered that she was unable to have children. So Elisha assured her that a miracle would take place in her life and she would have a baby within the next year.

You can tell how pained she is by her infertility because she says to Elisha, "No, my lord . . . Please, man of God, don't mislead your servant" (2 Kings 4:16). She might have been thinking, "Don't get my hopes up, Elisha. I can't take another disappointment. My heart can't be broken again."

If you or a loved one has dealt with infertility issues, then you know that it is a pain that runs deep within your soul. It doesn't go away. Life can be so difficult and painful. Often those of us who have had children simply cannot relate to that type of anguish that runs so deep. But certainly no couple in that situation wants someone playing games with their emotions. "Don't say we are going to have a baby in a year, Elisha," she might have thought. But sure enough, the lady has a child, "just as Elisha had told her" (2 Kings 4:17).

The boy grew. Everything was going great, until one day the dad and the boy were out in a field working. Life was perfectly normal, and then the boy said, "My head! My head!" (2 Kings 4:19).

I don't know what happened to this kid.

Was it a subarachnoid hemorrhage, like me? Maybe. It sounds like it. I said something similar on the day of my hemorrhage, when it felt like someone smashed me in the head with a Louisville slugger. I don't know what happened to this kid—I went to seminary, not med school. The dad knew it was serious—whatever it was—the dad knew this was bad. The Bible says, "His father told a servant, 'Carry him to his mother.' After the servant had lifted him up and carried him to his mother, the boy sat on her lap until noon, and then he died" (2 Kings 4:19-20).

What a horrible story.

It's heart-wrenching. This mom and dad had been waiting, waiting, waiting for a child, heartbroken because they couldn't have a baby, and then, miracle of miracles, they have a son. Joy of joys! No doubt he was lavished with love beyond measure. He's the apple of their eyes—their only son. Then following a sudden brain issue out in a field, he suddenly dies in his mother's arms.

If you have had to deal with the pain of the loss of a child, there is nothing more difficult, more tragic, more horrible. It's awful. Deep grief might not be labeled "chronic pain," but it is awful.

This story is one of my favorites not only because I can relate to the kid with really bad headache but also because the headache doesn't have the final word!

The story doesn't end with a funeral. No hearse drove to the scene.

To make a long story short, Elisha went to where the lifeless body of the boy was placed and prayed a prayer. God answered that prayer and the boy's life was restored. In fact, the Bible says, "The boy sneezed seven times and opened his eyes" (2 Kings 4:35).

Achoo! Achoo! Achoo! Achoo! Achoo! Achoo! Achoo! Alive! I don't know who was counting the sneezes, but the boy lived. It's my favorite story because it doesn't end with a headache.

Listen: your story need not end with your pain or "impossible" issues either. Elisha reminds us that God is bigger than any "impossible" situation.

God is mightier than your toughest foe.

God can handle your huge, massive mountain of troubles, all of your worries and heartaches, and your chronic pain. God can handle it.

BIBLICAL HELPS FOR THE CHRONIC PAIN SUFFERER

The Bible offers plenty of encouragement when health or emotions and life are getting you down.

For instance Exodus 2:24-25, though originally written to the enslaved children of Israel, speaks words of comfort and God's concern to anyone suffering: "God heard their groaning and he remembered his covenant with Abraham, with Isaac and with Jacob. So God looked on the Israelites and was concerned about them." The passage does not say anything about pain, but it sure is good to know that God hasn't forgotten us; he hears our prayers and knows what's going on. There have been plenty of "groaning" moments in this journey, and in every moment of suffering he is concerned.

In Deuteronomy when Moses was blessing the tribes, he said: "The eternal God is your refuge, and underneath are the everlasting arms" (33:27). Again, no mention of an ailment or remedies, but when we're suffering, isn't it reassuring to know that God is our refuge and that his everlasting arms are holding us up? I have relied on that passage frequently. While no one would confuse me with a "fire and brimstone preacher," there is no question when a headache is raging I'd rather be whispering than preaching. The only way I can preach (the *only* way) is because of God's everlasting arms holding me up and giving me strength.

The Psalms offer great assurances for the chronic pain sufferer. The reason so many people have memorized the 23rd psalm is because of the comfort offered in words like: "Even though I walk through the darkest valley, I will fear no evil, for you are with me; your rod and your staff, they comfort me" (verse 4). Sounds like Jesus is in my boat or (more accurately stated in the shepherd motif) in my pasture even when I'm walking through the messiest of pastures.

Psalm 42:11 says: "Why, my soul, are you downcast? Why so disturbed within me? Put your hope in God, for I will yet praise him, my Savior and my God." I might not be smiling in the storm, but I need not be in despair. Headache or any other ailment need not win the day. No matter how big the storm, God is bigger.

Moreover, I've read Psalm 121 in more hospital rooms and nursing homes than I can count. It continues to be such a great source of comfort when the psalmist proclaimed:

I lift up my eyes to the mountains—
where does my help come from?
My help comes from the LORD,
the Maker of heaven and earth.
He will not let your foot slip—
he who watches over you will not slumber;
indeed, he who watches over Israel
will neither slumber nor sleep.
The LORD watches over you—
the LORD is your shade at your right hand;
the sun will not harm you by day,
nor the moon by night.
The LORD will keep you from all harm—
he will watch over your life;

the LORD will watch over your coming and going
both now and forevermore.

Those words have offered comfort to the suffering for thirty centuries, and they still are relevant today. Our help is from the Maker of heaven and earth. He made you. Chronic pain is not beyond his specialty or his knowledge. He knows you and your issues.

Jesus offered powerful words of hope and encouragement in Matthew 11:

Come to me, all you who are weary and burdened, and I will give you rest. Take my yoke upon you and learn from me, for I am gentle and humble in heart, and you will find rest for your souls. For my yoke is easy and my burden is light. (Verses 28-30)

We are not a bother or a burden to him. On the contrary, Jesus told us to go to him when weary. In him, we will find our rest.

One of the by-products of my pain has been trouble sleeping. Getting a full night of solid sleep is very elusive. So the promise of finding our rest in him and discovering that our relief is through Christ has been a truth that I have held onto very tightly. I have claimed those words over and over again and as always Jesus has provided my rest.

Paul's words to the Romans are a great encouragement too, when he simply called the community of believers to: "Be joyful in hope, patient in affliction, faithful in prayer" (Romans 12:12). That's good advice no matter what ails you. When headaches or life get me down, the best treatment strategy contains Paul's big three: hope, patience, and prayer.

For me, the second attribute on Paul's short list has been the most difficult. I am usually hopeful. I try very hard to be faithful in prayer. But patience in affliction at times has been tricky. To get to that point, I have discovered it takes more than simply praying, "God, give me patience . . . *now*, please!" It's a daily, moment-by-moment matter of trust and obedience. It's saying, "I know God is at work. With all that I am, I know it, and I will trust him!"

The Bible might not directly list the seven healthy habits to battle headaches, gout, or back troubles, but God's Word is still a reassuring voice when the struggles of life are getting you down.

JESUS STILL CARES

In Matthew 14, Jesus himself was distressed. His cousin and a great man of God, John the Baptist, was murdered on the whim of a scorned woman. He was ready for some alone time to grieve and process all that was happening. But he didn't get solitude; crowds of people discovered Jesus and followed after him. Instead of saying something like, "Listen, you thoughtless miracle moochers, can't you give a guy a break? My cousin John has been killed. How about cutting me some slack? Is that too much to ask?"

But that conversation does not happen. Instead the Bible states, "When Jesus landed and saw a large crowd, he had compassion on them and healed their sick" (Matthew 14:14). Jesus was concerned for the hurting even as his own heart was hurting. As he observed the crowd, he had compassion.

I was just in a crowd of 110,000 people not long ago. The gathering of friends took place in Ann Arbor, Michigan. Of course, I am speaking of the University of Michigan Stadium (also known as "The Big House"). It's known as "The Big House" because on game day, more than 110,000 maize-and-blue-clad fans jam into the building to watch the Wolverines play football. As I looked around that stadium on a beautiful Saturday afternoon, some were yelling, some dancing, some sitting quietly, and some never sat throughout the entire game. I was reminded that Jesus died for every single one of those cheering fanatics. He would look over that crowd like the crowd in the first century and have compassion on them. His love is not thinned out by the volume of people or the color of their skin or the language they speak. (He even loves Ohio State Buckeye fans.) His love and compassion is great enough to include each person who has ever lived.

As such, I like to imagine Jesus looking over the crowded millions of chronic pain sufferers and responding in the same way—with compassion and healing. He's not preoccupied. He is not too busy. He doesn't measure pain as less worthy of divine intervention than cancer. He knows our struggles and our hurt. He sees, has compassion, and works in amazing ways.

"Working in amazing ways" does not always include a "boom! pain gone" type of miracle. But "working in amazing ways" does include giving strength to handle the pain. "Working in amazing ways" does include bringing hope in the midst of an episode and enabling one to help others in spite of the pain. There are plenty of "amazing workings" that God can do in your life without healing you of one particular ailment. Even if a miraculous physical healing does not occur in your life, that does not mean that God cannot work in amazing ways in your life.

THE PROMISE OF SCRIPTURE IS THAT IT'S NOT JUST ABOUT HERE AND NOW

Moreover, John the Revelator reminded us that there is coming a day when "God himself will be with them and be their God. 'He will wipe every tear from their eyes. There will be no more death' or mourning or crying or pain, for the old order of things has passed away" (Revelation 21:3b-4). A day is coming when your struggles will be over. What you are suffering through at this moment is not the end of the story. So hang in there, my fellow sufferers; according to God's Holy Word, our troubles will not last forever. God hears you, knows you, lifts you, and loves you! Jesus did not come to this earth so that you might experience a pain-free life. He came to this world so that you might experience him. He came so that you might experience a glorious hope throughout eternity. Those plans haven't changed for you. Pain or no pain, God has big plans for your future.

4 PAIN AND HEALING
ALMIGHTY GOD'S MIRACULOUS WORKING

Have you heard the old joke about the televangelist that taught his dog to speak? He called out "Speak, Fido! Speak!" And the dog immediately jumped to attention and barked, "Meow!" (Fido was "speaking in tongues." A dumb joke, I know.)

If you didn't like that joke, you'll probably hate this one. That same televangelist taught his dog to heel. He'd yell, "Heel, Fido! Heel!" and the dog would jump up on his hind legs, howl a couple of howls, and bop his paw on a stranger's forehead." (Grammatically, I should have written "Heal, Fido!" but that would have ruined the joke.) Okay, the jokes were already ruined. They were both poor attempts at humor. As you can obviously tell, my calling is not stand-up comedy. Phony televangelists and their dogs notwithstanding, the reality of healing is no joke. God still heals!

I've prayed for hundreds, if not thousands, of sick folks down through the years. You name the ailment, virus, or disease, and I've probably prayed for God to heal that particular disease or ailment.

I've prayed that God would knock the snot out of head colds.

And swat swine flu bugs back to the pigs of Timbuktu.

I've asked God to change mean, nasty, ugly cancer cells into happy, healthy, pretty cells.

I've prayed that hurting and broken bones would mend together.

I've anointed so many people with oil that I ought to have stock in the olive industry.

I've called upon God to step in so that no surgery was needed.

I've asked him to be in the operating room during surgery, after surgery, and throughout the entire recovery time.

I've requested that God would use medicines, doctors, nurses, technicians, and any other medical equipment or hospital personnel that might wander in the operating room during a procedure.

I guess I won't know until heaven (and then I probably won't care) just how many hospital rooms, emergency waiting areas, doctors' offices, and homes I've been in to pray with sick folks.

The point of all of this is that I am convinced that God still heals. I don't think for one second that all those prayers uttered were a waste of time. Oh, I might not believe in healing the way some white-suited televangelists do who at times, it would appear, are more intent on emptying people's wallets than emptying hospital corridors. Still I believe that *God* heals. I believe that just as Blind Bart (who was blind as a bat before he met Jesus, and then could see a gnat on a mongoose's nose after he met Jesus) was healed, people can be healed from what ails them today. God heals those afflicted physically, emotionally, spiritually, and every other way. Our God is a mighty healer.

James was not just exercising wishful thinking when he wrote: "Is anyone among you sick? Let them call the elders of the church to pray over them and anoint them with oil in the name of the Lord. And the prayer offered in faith will make the sick person well; the Lord will raise them up" (5:14-15). That passage is true, and I have quoted it in sermons and to sick folks probably as much as any verse in the Bible. Are you sick? Do you have pain issues? Call on the church to pray. Don't be afraid to be anointed with oil. Be anointed more than once if the problem persists. Hop in a vat of oil if you want to—just keep praying!

For all of our talk on prayer, books on prayer, and sermons on prayer, I think our real problem with prayer is that we spend too little time praying. I've known those who have complained about God not answering their prayers. All the while, I wonder if their prayers have been little more than lip service. Maybe our trouble isn't unanswered prayers but unuttered prayers. Could it be that our issues are not that God doesn't answer but that too often we haven't prayed? *A point of clarification:* I am not suggesting that if we pray hard enough or long enough or utter some magical word that God *is compelled* to heal us. I have no clue as to why some sick and needy are healed and why some sick and needy are not. Those decisions are above my pay grade. (I tell folks I'm in "sales" not "management" when it comes to the question of answered prayers.) Nor do I pretend to have the nature of intercessory prayer completely figured out. I've been praying for years, and I still don't know the exact nature of it all.

But this is what I know: God's Word tells us to pray for the sick and needy. And when we do pray, we trust that God Almighty knows exactly what is needed exactly when it is needed! As such, there are times when we are not healed in the manner we would prefer, but faith means saying, "I am still trusting God!" There are other times we may be like the lady in Mark 5 who had a bleeding disorder for twelve years; when she was healed, God said, in so many words, "Enough is enough. You've been sick long enough. No need for fancy words. No need for any other actions." And it's *boom*! Instantly healed! Go in peace!

In twenty-one centuries before Christ, God did the miraculous. Twenty-one centuries after Christ, God still does the miraculous!

So if something ails you today, pray on! Do you need a miracle today? Pray on! Today might be your day of healing. Today could be your day when God says about your issue, "Enough is enough." Boom! Healed! Go in peace!

I know God can heal people. I know it with everything that I am. I don't know why I was one of the 50 percent that survived a subarachnoid hemorrhage, but I believe it was God's healing touch upon me that enabled it. So read this: *God heals people.*

I really believe it. I believe that God can work such powerful miracles that doctors do a "Scooby Doo" double take while looking at an X-ray. I believe that God can make even the most hardened, empirically biased, scientifically minded, "show me the evidence" physicians scratch their heads and mutter to themselves, "I don't get it. I just don't get it." I believe that the same God who made lame guys walk still can. I believe the God who made once blind guys see still can! I believe the God who made diseases like leprosy disappear still has the power to do it! And I believe there is no chronic pain that has ever happened that is beyond God's ability to completely remove. God still heals!

Back in the 1970s, a musical opened on Broadway called *Your Arm's Too Short to Box with God: A Soaring Celebration in Song and Dance.* The musical was loosely based on the book of Matthew. Whatever you may think about the musical, I love the title. And for the pain sufferer, I think the play could be called, *Your Pain Is No Match for God.* Chronic pain and every other ailment are no competition for the Great Physician.

NOT EVERYBODY GETS HEALED ON PLANET EARTH

A world-renowned physician attends my church. He is an ear, nose, and throat specialist and has performed hundreds of delicate surgeries. I asked him how many times in his medical practice he witnessed a miracle—a "there is no other explanation but God's powerful working" type of miracle. He said, "Four times."

Four? Out of the hundreds (maybe thousands) of patients he has seen down through the years? Just four?

That's the problem. Four. Not four hundred. Not even forty. Just four.

No doubt the majority—maybe even all—of his patients had been prayed over by someone asking for a miracle. Some were healed through my friend's capable hands, and some were healed through medicines and treatments. But many weren't healed at all. Far more than four patients succumbed to their disease. Bottom line: God just doesn't physically heal everybody on this earth.

Why not?

I don't know. This book isn't trying to answer that question, because I don't know that answer. (See above comments about my pay grade.)

Here's what I do know—God is always with us. Do you remember all those verses quoted in the last chapter? I am convinced that Jesus is always in the boat during the storms. A story from my childhood illustrates exactly what I am talking about.

GOD IS WITH US IN THE STORMS

I used to love storms. I remember as a child seeing lightning flash across the sky and thinking it was the coolest thing. I loved to hear loud booming thunder too—the louder the better in my book. Storms were always more than okay. They were fun.

That's because I was viewing the storm from the safety of our house. I never worried. Our house could weather any storm. I live in Kansas now (we have real storms in Kansas—ever see *The Wizard of Oz?*), but I grew up in Michigan. It's the home of snowstorms but very few tornadoes and even fewer hurricanes. Rarely were storms frightening to me—except for one time.

My brother (also a preacher) and I have told this story over the years as one our family's most fearful moments. As a family, we would go camping. We had a pop-up camper. We would take our little Tradewinds tent-topped camper all across the country. When I was very young—four or five years old—we went to a campground somewhere. I think it was in Pennsylvania (I could be wrong—I was only four or five) and we began to set up our campsite.

No sooner had we begun setting up the campsite when we noticed the campground ranger going from campsite to campsite informing everyone of a major storm coming and that the prudent thing to do would involve going into a nearby town and getting a hotel room.

I don't know why my parents chose to stay and not heed the ranger's advice. Maybe they didn't want to spend the money on a hotel room. We were from Michigan, not Kansas. We know snow, not tornadoes. Maybe we were from a hardier (or more foolish) line of humanity than the others in the camp. I don't know what went into their decision-making process, but for whatever reason, we chose to hunker down for the night and weather the coming storm.

But that's not what made me afraid. Even when the rain started to fall and the thunder and the lightning started to occur, I was not afraid. For a four- or five-year-old kid, it was kind of fun. The camper was swaying and the rain was tap, tap, tapping. It was no big deal. There were loud booms of thunder. Cool! Bring it on! I liked thunder. It was fun.

I don't think my parents (especially my mom) thought it was an enjoyable experience. Looking back now, I am sure my parents' tension level was rising. Maybe they made a bad decision. Maybe they should have gotten a hotel room after all. Maybe deciding to stay in a pop-up camper during a tornado wasn't the wisest choice in their lives.

Oblivious to all of that, my brother and sisters and I started pestering one another. I know your families are perfect, but mine was not. We were in the closed, confined, canvas quarters of the camper; no one could go outside to play because of the storm. So we did the next best thing—we were taunting and teasing each other.

"Mom, Fred's picking on me."

"Dad, Beth has my sleeping bag."

"Ouch—Fred just gave me a hurtz donut."

"Not touching you, not touching you, not touching you."

That sort of thing.

Finally, my dad had had it. He was not a yeller. He was a pretty mild-mannered guy, but on that night, in the storm, in the dark, as the wind was blowing, the rain pouring, and the tension high—he got out of his bed and yelled out, "I've had it!" And he slammed the door.

Now, I was scared.

Everyone got quiet in the camper. My dad had left us. The storm was raging, and our dad was gone. He had never left us before, even when my older siblings (not me of course) behaved much worse. He never left us, but now when we needed his presence with this huge storm blowing, he was gone.

My sister Pam started singing the old hymn, "A Shelter in the Time of Storm." Maybe it brought her comfort to sing that hymn, but it didn't bring me any comfort at all.

I remember that was a long, long night. When I thought my dad was in the camper—no matter how bad the storm was blowing—I wasn't afraid. I knew my dad would take care of us. The storm didn't bother me a bit. Dad was there. Dad was tough. Dad was strong. But when I thought he was not in the camper, it was really scary.

Have you been there? *Why, God? Why?* There is a storm and you are not in the camper? I really need you now, but you have left me. When I need you the most, God, where are you? Have you asked those questions? That's a scary place, isn't it?

When we woke up the next morning I learned two very important lessons:

1. My dad really didn't leave us. He was in the camper the whole time. I just thought he left us, but he didn't. The door was rattling and he slammed it shut. It was so dark and the thunder so loud, I thought he left. But he didn't leave. He slammed the door and climbed back into bed. He didn't need to speak up anymore because at that point our entire sibling ribbing and taunts had stopped. He never knew that I was afraid or thought that he had left.

2. When we went outside, everybody else—literally everyone else in the campground—had left. We were the dumbest people in the campground—the only ones that stayed. There were trees uprooted. There were branches down. In fact, directly above our camper a huge branch had broken off of the tree, and in spite of the wind and rain, it did not fall on our camper. Which if it had, I'm not sure if I would be writing this story. Our family has always viewed that night as a night when God miraculously protected our family.

I tell you that story to say—just like my dad—God has not left you in your storm. Maybe you can't hear him. Maybe you can't see him. There are times when the storms we face are so loud and distracting that we don't hear the Savior's voice. Keep listening. You'll hear him. He has not and will not leave you.

HELP FROM ISAIAH AND A PSALM

The words in Isaiah 43 are still true:

But now, this is what the LORD says—
he who created you, Jacob,
he who formed you, Israel:
"Do not fear, for I have redeemed you;
I have summoned you by name; you are mine.
When you pass through the waters,
I will be with you;
and when you pass through the rivers,
they will not sweep over you.
When you walk through the fire,
you will not be burned;
the flames will not set you ablaze. (Verses 1-2)

Listen: bad things will come into your life. You will go through storms. Notice I didn't use words like *may* or *might* or *possibly could*. Storms *will* come. Problems *will* arise. There is going to be trouble in your life. Everybody has something. For me and millions of Americans, it's chronic pain.

Christians are not exempt from bad things happening, but the promise of God is that as his adopted child you are not alone. I love the good news of Psalm 34. It says: "The Lord is close to the brokenhearted and saves those who are crushed in spirit. The righteous person may have many troubles, but the Lord delivers him from them all" (verses 18-19). Even the righteous have troubles, but the Lord is close. He delivers. You can count on him.

A WEIRD THANKSGIVING PRAYER

On a Thanksgiving Sunday a couple of years ago, I instructed the folks in my congregation to take the quiet moments before participating in Communion to "count their blessings." Like the rest of the congregation, as the music was playing and as people were moving forward to receive the holy elements, I began to make a mental list of things to give thanks for. I was a set aback by the first thing that the Holy Spirit brought to my mind. It was not my salvation experience, or Karla and the boys, or my religious upbringing—all of which I am extremely thankful for—but rather the first item clearly in my mind in that moment was: headaches.

Headaches?! Are you kidding me? Thankful for headaches?

But that was my first thought, "Rob, are you thankful for your headaches?"

As I've written, headaches are my constant companion. That was the year I had had a migraine from April to August. While the Botox treatments greatly helped, my neurologist and I had not (and still haven't) gotten a complete handle on them. (I think I've become his star patient.) Even more than the brain hemorrhage year, that particular year I dealt with headaches on a constant, daily basis. Just a few months prior, I seriously considered taking a leave of absence from the church because of the daily and constant pain. It had been a horrible, horrible migraine stretch.

Quite honestly, here is what headaches did for me during that year—they caused me to take more drugs, have more IVs, get more injections, see more doctors, have my blood pressure taken more, spend more money, lose more sleep, eat less good food (thanks to the migraine diet), lose more weight, be more nauseated, spend more time in a dark, quiet room, and miss more evenings with the family than I cared to remember.

Here's what else the headaches did for me that year: they helped me pray more and trust God more. They made me more dependent upon God. I learned to look to him for my help and spend more time in his Word. Following the "Great Summer of the Migraine," I empathize with people better. Now I totally understand that all my strength is in God. There are times—lots of times—when I realize "all my strength is in God and if I am going to make it through the day, it will only be through his power and might." He is *always* faithful, and he has *always* come through *exactly* when I needed him. I had been able to endure through his power and might.

In other words, pain—for all of its stinkiness (not a word but you know what I mean—in all of its awfulness, terribleness, rottenness, and every other descriptor that I can use to describe the word *yuck*) has brought me closer to God and hopefully brought others closer to God too. So as strange as it might seem for me to type out these words, I am thankful for my headaches and the God who richly meets my needs in spite of those head boomers.

A PRAYER TO MAKE HABAKKUK PROUD

I'm not always where the prophet Habakkuk was as he concluded his little book, but I'm working on it. Habakkuk knew a thing or two about surviving, even thriving, in the middle of troubling times. I think I'm getting there. He wrote:

> Though the fig tree does not bud and there are no grapes on the vines, though the olive crop fails and the fields produce no food, though there are no sheep in the pen and no cattle in the stalls, yet I will rejoice in the LORD, I will be joyful in God my Savior. The Sovereign LORD is my strength; he makes my feet like the feet of a deer, he enables me to tread on the heights. (3:17-19)

A headache sufferer might rewrite Habakkuk's words this way: "Though my head feels like a drum and bugle corps is marching through my brain and there are no medicines that are taking the edge off, though the I'm sitting in a dark room and the house can't be quiet enough, though I'm sick to my stomach because of the pain, though I'm counting sheep but I can't seem to go to sleep, yet I will rejoice in the Lord, I will be joyful in God my Savior. The Sovereign Lord is my strength!"

Whether God heals me completely or whether I am healed when time shall be no more, I am convinced that God knows what is best for my life situation. I have learned that I can trust him. I want to rejoice in him and know that it is his strength (certainly not mine) that gets me through each and every moment.

Bible verses like Romans 8:28 are still true whether or not a migraine is booming. In that passage, Paul declared: "And we know that in all things God works for the good of those who love him, who have been called according to his purpose." God is working—even when we don't see it.

Even when the pain is raging, and the medicine isn't work-ing—God is still working. It's a matter of trusting that God is with me when skies are blue and all is well—but it doesn't stop there. God was with me when the brain hemorrhage occurred, and he is with me when the pain is raging.

While knowing that some good has come out of my chronic pain experience, please understand I don't quote Romans 8:28 because in some way I think my headaches are good. They are not good. I've tried to make the case that they stink. Really stink. I quote Romans 8:28 because of a belief that as headaches rage, God is still greater. God is still God. And at the end of time, in light of eternity, these "light and momentary troubles" (see 2 Corinthians 4:17) will be seen for what they were—light and momentary. In these troubles, God's grace became available and his peace came near. But they are not good, not fun, not something I would wish on my worst enemy.

REFLECTING JOSEPH'S ATTITUDE

I don't know whether or not Joseph of the Old Testa-ment experienced headaches. I know he experienced plenty of things that could give a guy a massive migraine. His jeal-ous brothers sold him into slavery; his father, Jacob, thought he was dead; he was a slave; he was falsely accused and spent time in prison.

All of those things we would rightly say were terrible. It's terrible when siblings don't get along; it's terrible when one is separated from an aging parent; it's terrible when the in-nocent are sent to prison. For years, a casual observer would have said Joseph was a good guy who had plenty of bad things happen to him. But that wasn't the end of the story.

Joseph's story ends as he is exonerated and sitting in the second most powerful seat in the most powerful empire in the world. He revealed his true identity to his brothers and he boldly declared, "You intended to harm me, but God intended it for good to accomplish what is now being done, the saving of many lives" (Genesis 50:20).

At any time during all of those terrible experiences for Joseph, no one would have questioned him for shouting out loud, "Hey, what's going on here! I didn't deserve any of this junk in my life!" But at any of those points along the way, he would not have been seeing the big picture. He would not have seen how God used all of those experiences to make him into the man he would become. He couldn't have seen how he would be held in high regard in the most powerful country in the world. He could not have imagined how he would be a blessing to the nation and to his family.

The point: I can't think of a good reason to delay my healing from chronic pain. It is certainly my desire to be pain free. I'd love to be able to eat a taco without knowing that forty-five minutes later I will be stricken with a massive headache. I'd love to be able to listen to the weather guy on TV say "there's a storm front coming in" without in the back of my head hearing, "There is a massive migraine coming in." I wish all of that would go away. But I also know I don't have all of the details. I don't have all of the facts. I don't see everything God sees. I don't know how God is going to use all of these experiences, but I believe God will use these experiences for his glory—even if that is simply in my being able to express glory to him in a more complete manner.

PAUL'S PERSPECTIVE

Just last night I was working on this book. It had been my "pincushion day," the day I received my quarterly Botox. I also was experiencing a medium-level headache. Karla looked over at me and said, "I sure hope you finish that book and are able to help people with pain so that God can then heal you."

I think she was thinking like Paul in 2 Corinthians. Paul explained to the suffering believers in Corinth that God "comforts us in all our troubles, so that we can comfort those in any trouble with the comfort we ourselves receive from God" (1:4). I think that was Karla's point. Through my experiences, others might be helped.

I hope she is right. My continued prayer is that you are helped as you read this book or hear my story. But the truth is I don't know that God is waiting until this book is published to heal me. I don't know that the delay in relief is to make me better, stronger, smarter, more patient, or give me any other wonderful attribute. I don't know if I will ever be completely healed from headaches—that's not the point. God knows more than me. (That statement was the most ridiculously understated sentence in any book of all time. Of course, God knows more than me.) Still, I know this: my purpose in life is not to simply live and be happy. My purpose is not even to live a migraine-free life. My purpose is to bring glory to God, and if God gets more glory through a migraine-full preacher than a migraine-free preacher, may the name of the Lord be praised.

As a preacher of the gospel, I hope that my trials (as much as I have hated them at times) can point people to Christ. And quite frankly, if some people are helped (or better yet—come to Christ) in part through this book or through my ministry or through living a faithful life in the midst of headaches, then their salvation has far superseded the minor troubles I have experienced. Are you kidding me? It's not even close. I hope people see Jesus in me in the midst of my pain. In spite of it, I want those that observe my life to say, "Wow, look how God is being lifted in the midst of such pain!"

The same is true for you. Are you living to bring glory to God? Even with chronic pain, are you bringing glory to God? The pain will not last forever. Keep striving to glorify the Lord whether you are in pain or all is well.

5 | PAIN AND PRAYER
ASKING FOR PHYSICAL RELIEF

I don't know what makes a person a great prayer. Is it just that the person's prayers are answered in a powerful, glorious way? Is that the sole determining factor—or should I have written the "soul" determining factor? If someone is gifted in praying, does that mean that all of his or her prayers are heard by God with the same intensity? If someone connects with the Almighty and has a supernatural encounter, wouldn't that be indicative of being a great prayer even if the request is not answered in the manner that the prayer intended?

I've learned that when my head is pounding, I pray a lot. I wish I could say that I pray just as much when my head is pounding as I do when it isn't pounding, but honestly, that's not the case. I pray more with a headache. Mostly, I pray more because when I have a massive, in-a-dark-room, no-noises type of headache, all I can do is pray. Does the headache always go away when I pray? Nope. In fact, of all the headaches that I have had and of all the time I have prayed for God to "make it go away," I can't recall any time when it instantly vanished. There has never been a "Boom!

Done!" moment for my headaches. Still, when I am praying with a headache—even when I am praying for others when my head is hurting—it seems that I am closer to God.

I wish I could write that I am just as close to God when all is well. I wish I could say that my prayers have the same intensity—headache or no headache. But they just don't. What that indicates about my spiritual state I am not exactly sure—I'm just keeping it real. I think it's similar to what athletes say about playing in a big game. They are focused and "dialed in" for all the games, but in the big games, most athletes will admit to being particularly focused. They concentrate a little more. They are more aware of the smallest details of preparation. For me, when a headache is raging, I am more keenly aware of my senses. Noise is louder. Lights are brighter. I think all of my senses are heightened.

My spiritual sense is heightened too. I pray with a greater urgency. I am focused on what God might be saying at that moment. I am listening with a better spiritual ear.

I wish I were more like some of the great prayer warriors in the Bible. There are a lot of people gifted in praying in the Bible. People prayed mighty prayers, and God answered those prayers in impressive fashion. And apparently they didn't have chronic pain when they were praying.

Take a look at Moses, for example. No doubt he prayed some great prayers, full of confidence and faith, as he led the people of Israel for those forty years. Joshua was strong and courageous. He met with God. He had a pretty open communication line with the Almighty too.

Daniel was a great prayer. The guy prayed three times a day before getting tossed into the den as the lions' lunch buffet. Shadrach, Meshach, and Abednego had to have prayed some pretty hot prayers in the fiery furnace. There are also plenty of examples in the New Testament of great people of prayer.

A WRESTLING CHAMPION
(A PRAYER WRESTLING CHAMPION)

But if I had my choice, I would want to be like praying champion Epaphras!

E-what, or is it E-who?

E-paphras! He is a "who," not a "what."

When I was on a mission trip to Swaziland, I had the opportunity to preach. I was going over my sermon with the well-educated man who was going to translate the sermon for me. Preaching in another culture is always a little difficult. Certain words communicated in one culture don't always communicate the same thing in another culture. So we were going over the sermon to make sure everything "worked." As we looked over the words, we got to a spot in the sermon where I was planning on using an illustration that I thought would work in any culture. It was a story about Tiger Woods. Everybody in the world knows Tiger Woods, right? I said to him, "Will the people in the congregation know who Tiger Woods is?" (Thinking if there is anyone on the entire planet that everyone knows, it's Tiger Woods.) The translator said (and I quote), "*What* is Tiger Woods?" Not *who* is Tiger Woods? "What?" I chose to not use that illustration.

Epaphras is a "who." He is a very important "who"—a man of God—and "what" he did is pray.

Epaphras doesn't get a lot of print in God's Word, but he is a hero of mine. My heroes growing up were Al Kaline in baseball, Barry Sanders in football, and Gordie Howe in hockey, but when it comes to prayer, it's Epaphras hands down. The dude was the type of prayer that I want to be.

Epaphras is mentioned once in Philemon and in exactly two verses in Paul's letter to the Colossians. It's at the end of his epistle to the church. Paul is wrapping up the letter, and, like at the end of a children's Christmas musical when the program director receives a box of chocolates and proceeds to thank all of the moms and dads who helped put the production together, Paul mentioned all the different people that had been helping him while under house arrest in Rome. These are people that the church folks at Colossae would also have known. Paul wrote this: "Epaphras, who is one of you and a servant of Christ Jesus, sends greetings. He is always wrestling in prayer for you, that you may stand firm in all the will of God, mature and fully assured. I vouch for him that he is working hard for you and for those at Laodicea and Hierapolis" (Colossians 4:12-13).

"He is always wrestling in prayer for you."

Epaphras was a prayer wrestling hero. He was not a phony pro wrestler type with a stage name like "Epaphras the Crazy-eyed Collision from Colossae," pumped up and ready to rip telephone books in two. He was more like an Olympic prayer wrestling champion—driven, intense, and compelled by a never-quit-praying attitude.

Far from an Olympic wrestler (or pro wrestler, for that matter), I did a little wrestling in high school. No one will ever confuse me with a wild-eyed champion. I had no nickname. I wrestled in the 105-pound weight division. At the time, I actually weighed about 95 pounds (if I had a lot of loose change in my pockets and a lot of heavy clothes on), but I didn't wrestle as a 98-pounder (the lowest weight class at the time) because the reigning 98-pounder of my high school could easily twist me into a pretzel. He was a monster—well, as much of a monster as a 98-pound high school sophomore could be. I thought I had a better chance wrestling at 105 pounds. So I never had to lose weight to get to 105 pounds—I just had to lose my dignity wearing the wrestling unitards and lose my pride as I often found myself with my back on the mat as the referee slammed his hand on it. (Other schools in my conference had 105-pound "monsters"—I guess I didn't consider that possibility.)

I wrestled enough to know that it's hard work. It takes discipline and determination. All the wrestlers I know mean business. The wrestlers that won had a resolve that would not quit. Surrender was not in their vocabulary. Even when twisted and in an awkward, painful position, they wouldn't quit. They would keep at it—working, thinking, and trying to put a move on their opponent that would turn the match over in their favor. They would never stop until the referee slapped his hand on the mat, indicating that the wrestling match was over, or until the buzzer had sounded, indicating time was up.

The Colossae homeboy Epaphras was that type of prayer. Like a champion wrestler, I picture him (not in a unitard— that would be weird) as a guy who prayed and prayed and didn't stop praying. As a guy "who wrestled in prayer," I imagine he went before the Lord, kept going to the Lord, sought the Lord, kept seeking after God, prayed on his own behalf, and prayed also on behalf of his family and friends.

Think of him as a tag-team prayer wrestler. Back in my days of watching big-time wrestling, occasionally wrestlers would team up against another pair of wrestlers. Instead of one wrestler versus another, in a tag-team wrestling match it would be two wrestlers fighting against another pair. Only one could be on the wrestling mat at a time. The way for the nonparticipating wrestler to get in on the action on the mat was to tag hands with his partner. Hence, the name for this type of match is "tag team." I think Epaphras's friends would tag him with their requests, knowing he was a prayer wrestling champ.

"Epaphras, could you pray for my kids?" Tag.

"You got it."

"Epaphras, could you pray for my relationship with my wife?" Tag.

"You got it."

"Epaphras, we are going to have a tough conversation with a nonbeliever. Could you pray?" Tag.

"You got it."

That's what prayer wrestling champions do. They pray and keep praying and don't stop praying. When situations looked bad, he prayed. When trials or trouble were brewing, he prayed. When it seemed like the enemy was winning and he was on his back and the referee was about to slap the mat, he continued to wrestle in prayer. When it looked like time was running out and the clock was ticking down on a particular matter, he kept on praying. That's what prayer wrestling champions do. He put the situations of life into a headlock—he wrestled in prayer!

When you are battling pain, that's what you need to be—an Epaphras-like world champion prayer wrestler. Keep on praying. Don't stop praying. Don't allow life or circumstances or what the shouting crowd is saying to get you off focus or a pain in the cranium to cause you to stop—just keep on praying. Put that pain in a prayer "headlock." Be a prayer wrestling champion. Of course, the best-case scenario is when you have another Epaphras-like prayer that is willing to be your tag team member. A person you can go to and say,

"Today is a rough day." Tag.

He or she responds, "I'm on it. I'm praying."

If you are thinking, "I am not a champion of anything—especially when I'm in pain. Wrestling champions are strong and athletic. They are fierce and competitive. They look nothing like me when I am in pain."

Okay. How about looking like a weak and helpless widow. Could you look like that?

A CHAMPION THAT DOESN'T LOOK LIKE A CHAMPION

The widow Jesus described in Luke 18 was an Epaphras-type woman of prayer. And she looked nothing like a wrestling champion. I'm sure she didn't feel like the "Crazy Colossian Prayer Champion," but she had the same determination and the same never-quit attitude. She might not have looked like a champion, but she was one.

The story in Luke 18 begins this way: "Then Jesus told his disciples a parable to show them that they should always pray and not give up" (verse 1).

It's like we are at the corner of the mat and are about to hear the advice of the Great Prayer Wrestling Coach motivating a tired prayer wrestler.

Jesus is saying, "Come in close, boys—I've got an important lesson for you. When you are facing a tough foe and you are tempted to give up; when you are praying for the pain to go away and it's still there; when you are saying, 'What's the use, I've prayed a thousand times for this pain to end and it never has—why pray?' Then hear this."

Before we get to Jesus' story, let me ask you—have you been there?

Has your pain gotten you to the point where you have prayed and prayed and prayed and nothing seems to be happening? And you are tempted to say, "What's the use?" Believe me, I've been there. Like when I was a high school non-wrestling champion, maybe you feel that you are not prayer wrestling material. You are on your back and the referee is raising his hand to slap the mat. You're thinking, "I'm done." Are you feeling that way?

Hold on. Don't stop. Don't quit. Don't throw in the towel. Don't give up. Don't ever give up. Listen to this reminder from Jesus:

He said: "In a certain town there was a judge who neither feared God nor cared what people thought. And there was a widow in that town who kept coming to him with the plea, 'Grant me justice against my adversary.'

"For some time he refused. But finally he said to himself, 'Even though I don't fear God or care what people think, yet because this widow keeps bothering me, I will see that she gets justice, so that she won't eventually come and attack me!'" (Luke 18:2-5)

The story revolves around a widow. Usually, I don't envision a widow as a great wrestling champion. In my mind, the widow is old, feeble, and probably could not fight her way out of a wet paper bag. My guess is she could not tell the difference between a headlock and a half nelson. (Truth be told—I couldn't tell you the difference between those wrestling moves either.) It's probably stereotypical to think of her only in terms of a little old lady, but I think that was the message Jesus was trying to convey. He didn't say, "In a certain town there was a big tough guy who happened to have a little trouble." No, it was a widow—a poor, troubled widow. She was on the bottom of the pecking order. On the lowest rung of society, she was a helpless widow. But this widow is different. She is tough!

Being a widow is never easy—not in the first century or in the twenty-first century. My mom is a widow, and I remember the first several months after my dad passed away were not easy for her at all. My dad's illness was not very long, and when he passed away it was an abrupt change for my mom. She had relied on my dad for many things. For example, she hadn't pumped her own gas in her car in years. It was just one of the things my dad always did. I'm not sure if they even had self-service gas stations the last time she had put gas in the car. But now, dad was gone and life was different—in things much more serious than filling up a tank with gas. Everything changes when you are a widow.

Being a widow in the Middle East two thousand years ago was especially difficult. When Jesus told this story, a widow in the first century generally had no education, no job, no money, no property, no status—nothing. There was no social security, no retirement plan, and no Medicare. No open enrollment supplement plans. No disability parking privileges. No senior citizen discounts. No government bailouts. No social agencies or senior citizen advocacy groups. No AARP. No help. If she had family who could take her in or who could provide for her, then she would probably endure. If not, she might have to become a beggar—the first-century equivalent to a bag lady—a social outcast. This lady did not have a bright future.

But this poor widow had another problem that would only compound her problems and further complicate her life. She also had an "adversary." We don't know exactly who this person was—that's not the point. The point is somebody was bothering and harassing her. Maybe this adversary was intimidating her physically and pushing her around. Maybe the adversary was the town gossip and a rumormonger who was spreading all sorts of untruths and lies about the widow. Maybe this adversary was a crook and was stealing the few possessions that she had. There is no telling who this adversary might have been or what the adversary was doing. All we know is that there was a person in her life that was making her daily existence extremely problematic.

From her response to the judge, it certainly appears that the adversary was winning and she was losing in this first-century tussle. She needed justice. But where could she get justice? The widow had no way to protect herself, no relatives to help, no government agency that was about to step in and offer relief. She only had one shot to get rid of this scoundrel, and it meant going before a known crooked judge, hoping that he would take up her cause. (Read: fat chance!)

She stood alone before this uncaring judge. She didn't have a lot of choices. No hot-shot lawyer was offering any pro bono work. What else could she do? She went before the judge by herself.

Jesus describes this judge in very unflattering terms. He did not fear God. He did not care about his fellow humans. Of all the judges in the land, this guy would probably have been the last judge anyone would want to have presiding over a case. If I'm in trouble, I want a godly judge who understands that there is a greater Judge watching, or at least I'd want a moral judge who cares at least a little bit for the people in his courtroom. No one will confuse this guy with King Solomon or Judge Judy. What this judge lacked in godliness, he made up for with an equal lack of humanitarian concern. That's some judge! How did he get to be a judge in the first place?

Without fearing God, he had no one to whom he was accountable. It goes without saying—if he believes he is not accountable to God and doesn't fear God, then he probably doesn't respect God's Word. He doesn't think about the fact that one day there will be a time of reckoning when he will stand before another Judge, the greatest Judge, and give an account of his decisions. He doesn't comprehend that one day as an earthly judge he will be standing before a holy, heavenly Judge. If you are a judge who doesn't fear God or recognize that a day of judgment is coming, you make up your own rules and play the game as you want to play it with little regard for the eternal consequences. Justice and morality are only based on what will suit your fancy. Did I mention this was the worst judge you could possibly stand before?

Without respect for people, this judge didn't care how his decisions affected those who were looking for justice or mercy. He didn't see the people coming before him as victims or fellow citizens or people who have been given a tough time in life, and certainly he did not view them as brothers and sisters. He saw them as problems, bothers, and headaches, so to speak. More than likely, if you are a judge who doesn't fear God or doesn't care about your fellow humans, you are out to enrich only yourself or gain greater position in the mind of the society's movers and shakers. People like the widow—people with little status and even fewer financial resources—are not the way to move up to the next rung of the social ladder; they are a bother at best and a trap to actually move down the ladder at worst.

So where does this poor widow stand? No money. No influence. No strings to pull. No political clout. No secretly taken pictures of the judge's improprieties that she can use for a blackmail scheme. What in the world could she do to influence this crooked judge?

It makes you want to cry out to her, "Don't waste your time. This judge (as messed up as he is) is probably in cahoots with that person who is hassling you. He's only out for what he can get. You don't have anything he wants. You have no leverage over him. He'll laugh in your face. He'll kick you out of his courtroom. He won't listen. He doesn't dish out mercy. He won't offer justice. You are in a hopeless situation. He won't care about you."

In Jesus' story, that's pretty much how the unmerciful judge responded and how her situation was going. "For some time he refused" (Luke 18:4).

I am not sure how long "some time" is, but I think it was a while, which makes this widow all the more special. Did I mention she has a little Epaphras in her? Like a prayer wrestling champion, she didn't give up easily. When knocked down, she brushed herself off, picked herself up, and said, "I'm going back into the match! I'm going to face that crooked, messed-up judge. I've not been knocked out. I'm still kicking. I'm still scrapping. I've got no other options or choices. If that judge is the only judge in town, then he is going to see my side of this conflict one way or another." Sounds like a wrestling champion from Colossae. "Quit" was not in her vocabulary. She would not stop or be kept down by this crooked judge—even as he ignored her "for some time."

But how could she keep going back? What would be different the next time she returned to stand before the judge? She doesn't sound like the blackmailing type even if she had some juicy evidence of impropriety. She didn't have anything to hold over this judge. (Remember: he didn't fear God or care about his fellow humans.) Bribe him? With what? She is a poor widow. What could she say in hearing two or hearing three that she didn't say in the first hearing before the judge? What could possibly make this judge change his mind?

Somewhere along the line, she came up with a game plan. It was a winning strategy when facing a loser of a judge. She thought, "I know what I'll do. I'm going to pester this guy. I'm going to be wherever he goes. He is going to see my face whenever he turns around. I'm going to sit in his courtroom. I'm going to follow him home. When he is working out in the gym, I'll be there. When he goes to the market, I'll bag his groceries. When he grabs a coffee at the Jerusalem Java House, I'll offer him milk and sugar. This judge won't be able to turn around without seeing my troubled face. He'll start seeing me in his dreams."

Today he would have filed a restraining order against her. We would call this lady a stalker. Maybe we would think she is a little too obsessed with her plight. "Can't you take 'no' for an answer?" someone might ask.

This lady was undeterred by the crooked judge. She would not stop showing up in his courtroom until, in one way or another, the judge would do the right thing. And here's the crazy thing: it worked. She pestered and pestered and pestered the corrupt judge until one day he said, "I can't take it anymore. This crazy lady is driving me bananas! Somebody take care of that adversary of hers!"

So the story ends with the crooked, thoughtless, terrible, unfaithful judge finally giving in to the widow's request—not because of kindness, goodwill, or a sense of justice welling up within him, but because this lady had a tremendous ability to pester and be a bother and get under his skin. She became the patron saint of nags and annoying pests everywhere. She's a little creepy, but at least she got what she wanted.

Now remember Jesus told this story so that "we would pray and not give up." And if you stop reading the story right there, you might make the entirely wrong conclusion. You might think, "Well, we must be the like the poor, crazy, half-creepy widow. No status. No connections. We are unable to handle our life's problems on our own, and we probably need to be a tad obsessive. And God must be the judge. He's busy. He's kind of mean. He's not really interested in our situation—he has a universe to run and harps to build and heavenly mansions to construct and golden road construction crews to manage and angels' Union 777 to keep in line. God is much too important to bother with my situation or my kids or my job or my headache. It's best not to inconvenience him unless my dilemma is *really* important." But if it is *really* important, and if we are desperate enough, we can always do what the creepy, crazy widow did. Just pester the snot outta him. Spend hours on our knees. Get our friends to pester him too. The more the merrier. And sooner or later, if we keep bothering him long enough, if we keep sitting in his courtroom, we might just wrestle a blessing out of the Judge of the universe. Eventually he'll shout, "Okay! Enough already! I can't take it anymore! Will somebody take care of that pesky pastor's (in my case) or that lunatic lawyer's or that overbearing computer operator's situation?"

Does that sound right to you? Does that sound like a loving heavenly Father to you? I sure hope not.

I've talked to people—usually in desperate situations—who have been praying and praying, and they are looking for some magic word or secret formula that will finally, oh so finally, get God to act on their behalf. In their twisted theology, God is like that judge—not really doing anything to help and maybe even a little mean. So they resort to pestering him like nobody's business and they think that maybe, just maybe, he will eventually work on their issues. If they persist long enough, if they are annoying enough, stalking enough, or irritating enough, then God will get tired of hearing their voices, and he will finally relent.

I hope it goes without saying: that is some bad, bad theology! Jesus himself went on to tell us that this is not the way to interpret this story.

And the Lord said, "Listen to what the unjust judge says. And will not God bring about justice for his chosen ones, who cry out to him day and night? Will he keep putting them off? I tell you, he will see that they get justice, and quickly." (Luke 18:6-8)

Listen: we are not like the widow. Not at all. She was poor, powerless, forgotten, and half-crazy. Brothers and sisters, that is not you! We are children of the King! We are in God's family. We don't have to search for some magic word or secret formula—we can approach him and say, "Hello, Father, it's your boy, Rob. Can we talk? I have been having these headaches, and . . ." There is no need for perfect words. No need to use King James English when you pray. Just be open, honest, and true. He hears you. The first time you prayed and the last time you prayed and every prayer in between he has heard. He has heard every single word. And he loves you!

By the way, it's not like you are informing God of a situation that he is unaware of or has turned a blind eye to. He knows your situation. God knows about every single migraine and every single headache that I have ever experienced in my entire life. I am not cluing him in to the situation in my prayers. He is not making me wait for an answer simply for the sake of waiting. Hopefully, my prayers are drawing me to a closer intimacy with the Father who loves me and cares deeply for my ultimate joy.

That's the point. God is nothing like the rotten judge in Jesus' story. The judge was uncaring, preoccupied, a real jerk—but our God is righteous, holy, trustworthy, loving, and kind. He is "Our Father which art in heaven" (Matthew 6:9, KJV). He is not the rotten, uncaring, unresponsive King of heaven. Don't think that you have to pester, pester, pester to get some kind of positive response out of God—he loves you. He really loves you. Is that how you treat the people you love? Turn them into stalkers and people who nag and beg and pester? No. You would wrap your arms around them. You would remind them of your strength and your presence. You would whisper in their ear, "Hold on. I'm here. No worries." That is exactly what God will do for you!

JESUS' LOVE AND UNANSWERED PRAYERS

In another place, Jesus said this:

Ask and it will be given to you; seek and you will find; knock and the door will be opened to you. For everyone who asks receives; the one who seeks finds; and to the one who knocks, the door will be opened.

Which of you, if his son asks for bread, will give him a stone? Or if he asks for a fish, will give him a snake? If you, then, though you are evil, know how to give good gifts to your children, how much more will your Father in heaven give good gifts to those who ask him! (Matthew 7:7-11)

Someone might say, "I've read those verses. I've claimed them a few times even. But I've had a few situations down through the years where I've prayed and prayed and prayed, and God didn't answer. So what's the deal? I was knocking but no doors were opened. No help came. I've been asking for bread and fish, but it feels like I've been given stones and snakes. Where are all the good things promised?"

That's the real question, isn't it?

We want to believe that God is not like the crooked judge. When everything is going well in our lives—we don't have a sick or wayward kid or we don't have massive pain or any real troubles at that particular moment—we say: "Yea, God's not like that crooked judge at all. Ask and it will be given to you."

But when we've been praying and praying and staying up all night wondering and worrying about a situation with a child or a grandchild, or when the pain is there and has been there for a few months, and God seems to be pretty silent, it's tough. It sure seems that our prayers are like giant spiritual-sounding boomerangs—we throw out the words in the direction of the sky and they just keep coming right back to us. It's easy to begin to wonder and ask: "What's the deal,

God? Why pray? I've been asking but nothing has been given to me. What's the deal? Why am I spending this time on my knees? If I am not required to pester or stalk you with prayer requests, then why aren't you responding? How about a 'Boom! Healed! Done!' type of word out of you, Lord?"

Have you been there? If you have not been there, you will be there someday.

It's natural when you have chronic pain to pray like crazy, to have faith that God will miraculously and powerfully remove it. But what happens when he doesn't?

I've had friends who believed if they had enough faith—faith the size of a mustard seed—a mountain would move. Quite frankly, they didn't want to see Mount Everest move one hundred feet to the left—they just wanted their loved one well. They had faith. They prayed. And it didn't happen. Mountains didn't move. No miracle cure came. Nothing. Then, these faith-questioning people came and said to me, "Pastor, *why didn't it happen?* Why pray? God says, 'Seek.' I sought, but nothing good happened."

Now I think I know the theological answer. I think. The theological answer seems to be that I don't want God to abandon his sovereignty at my prayer time. God is sovereign before I pray, and God is sovereign after I pray. God knows and does the absolute best—always. There is no viable alternative candidate for "Lord of the Universe" than the one we have. If God doesn't work a miracle, then a miracle wasn't what was needed at that moment. I get all of that.

But what do you say when that brokenhearted parent or that worried spouse or that troubled student has a lot more questions than answers? Or how do you explain it to yourself when you are dealing with pain that is there day after day after day? You want to say, "I've prayed and prayed, and

I don't know what else to do. Why doesn't God just end this whole ordeal?"

Again, why did Jesus tell us this parable? What did Luke say? Jesus told them this parable "to show them that they should always pray and not give up" (Luke 18:1). So the parable's point—as I've just explained—is that we are not like the widow, but rather we are a child of the King. God is not like the crooked judge, so we don't have to pester, pester, pester him—he is our loving Father. Still, Jesus said: keep on praying, don't give up. Don't pester, but keep on praying.

Is that a contradiction? I don't think it is.

PRAYING DIFFICULT PRAYERS

The answer is in praying difficult prayers. Praying is not cluing God in to your situation. He already knows. Praying is not convincing God that your particular pain is really bad—again, he already knows. Praying is not pestering God until he finally relents. Praying is recognizing God loves us, knows best, and is in control. Prayer is recognizing that we can trust him even (especially) in the middle of our troubling circumstances.

That's the tricky part of prayer—trusting when we don't see the outcome. Trusting when the answer we'd like doesn't seem to be coming. Telling God the problem is not hard. That's easy. People (even nonbelievers) do it all the time:

"My kid is sick!"

"My dad is in trouble."

"I need a job."

"My situation is bad."

"I have pain that will not quit."

It's easy to pray the problem—it doesn't take much effort to let God know what's going on in our life or to ask God for things. Sit in the majority of "prayer meetings" during request time, and you will think that Christian folk are the unhealthiest and most problem-filled people on the planet. Most of our requests involve physical needs. But is that all prayer is? I know this is a book about dealing with a physical ailment, but even the chronic pain sufferer need not relegate prayer to only being about his or her pain.

Here's what is hard to pray: "Lord, here's the problem. I have massive pain. I know you are at work even when I don't see much going on, and Lord, you know my heart's desire, but I want your heart's desire (and here comes the kicker) even if that is not my heart's desire."

That's a difficult prayer to pray, and after it's been prayed, the prayer time can move on to other more pressing needs like the nonbelieving next door neighbor or the ungodly influences in society.

Praying a tough prayer with major pain is holding on to the faithfulness of God even when the evidence of our long-awaited answer is not around. Praying a difficult prayer is submitting to the sovereignty of God even when it might be contrary to our wishes and desires.

It's Job praying, "Naked I came from my mother's womb, and naked I will depart. The LORD gave and the LORD has taken away; may the name of the LORD be praised" (Job 1:21). He prayed that prayer after he lost everything. Everything.

It's the Old Testament captives in Babylon saying in faith, "Next year, Jerusalem," even though they had said those words every year for decades. Like Chicago Cubs fans at the end of the baseball season, the captives said, "Wait until next year." Only the captives' circumstances were much more significant than a century of losing baseball.

It's Jesus praying in the garden: "Father, if you are willing, take this cup from me; yet not my will, but yours be done" (Luke 22:42). That's praying hard.

It's not giving up. It's becoming a prayer wrestling champion like Epaphras and the widow. It's not giving in. It's being convinced that even if the referee is about to slap the mat or the judge keeps saying no, if we are still breathing and kicking, the fight isn't over.

Prayer trusts that God is on the throne and that you can approach him. You are his child. You can go before him with your confusion, hurts, questions, anxiety, worries, and doubts. In the midst of your struggle, it's allowing God to grab you in his arms and hear him say, "I'm here. You're going to make it. Don't give up. You just see a little bit, I see the whole deal. You see the moment. I see eternity. I know this is a really big deal to you, but I will give you the strength to see it through. I can handle it."

It's learning the truth of William B. Walford's words. You may not know his name, but you may have sung his song. He wrote these words:

Sweet sixty seconds of prayer!
Sweet sixty seconds of prayer!
That calls me from the world of care.

Wait a minute (pun intended)—it's not sweet sixty seconds of prayer. That's what we do too often—pray for about sixty seconds (if that). But the song says:

Sweet hour of prayer,
Sweet hour of prayer,
That calls me from a world of care.

The line I like best:

In seasons of distress and grief
My soul has often found relief,
And oft escaped the tempter's snare
By thy return, sweet hour of prayer!

That's praying hard—in those seasons of distress and grief, still going before the Holy One. It's saying, "Lord, here's the deal." Then you lay out all of those burdens that are weighing heavy on your heart. Praying is not pestering. It's saying, "Here's my desire, but more than my desire, more than my plan, more than what I think is best, I want your desire. I want what you *know* is best, and in the meantime, Lord, in my season of distress and grief—my soul *desperately* needs to find relief. More than pain relief, I want you. I want more of you. I want to be so close to you that there is never a doubt of who is holding my hand through these trials."

That's why we need to pray!

PRAYER AS THE FIRST RESPONSE— NOT THE LAST RESORT

I was copied in on an email. It was written from one friend to another. The first friend has cancer. It doesn't look good. There are lots of problems, lots of bad reports, lots of sadness. The second friend was writing a letter of encouragement. It was a nice and encouraging letter (so all in all, mission accomplished). Now, I don't want to be too critical, and I understand the intent of the letter. But "Friend No. 2" concluded the email with these words: "I will be praying for you . . . I wish I could do more."

"I wish I could do more"? Do more than pray? Do more? Is that possible? What more can you do but go before God Almighty and present your requests? If we really believe that God is in control, and we really believe that we can have an audience through prayer with the Creator and Giver of Life, what more can we do? There is absolutely nothing *more* that we could possibly do. Everything else will be secondary to that first calling of prayer.

Prayer should be our first response, not our last resort. It is not an attitude that says, "Ugh, I might as well pray—I can't do anything else." Prayer is going on the offense. It's proactive. It's the greatest and most effective weapon we have in dealing with the pains and struggles of life. Prayer is the key to victory.

I wish my friend would have concluded the letter by saying: "I'm praying for you—and if there are any lesser things that I can do for you, I'll do that too!"

Please know whatever you're facing, whatever trials may come, whatever burdens you are trying to bear, take them to the Lord in prayer. It's not the last-ditch effort—it should be the first call to action. Paul said it this way to his young apprentice Timothy: "I urge you, *first of all*, to pray for all people. Ask God to help them; intercede on their behalf, and give thanks for them" (1 Timothy 2:1, NLT, italics mine). First of all, let's pray!

Why pray for that pain, even though you've prayed a thousand times before? Jesus says to pray. In fact, Paul tells us to "pray continually" in 1 Thessalonians 5:17. You and every person you know need someone to be a "Crazy-Eyed Colossian Prayer Wrestling Champion" like Epaphras—wrestling in prayer, not stopping no matter what the time clock says or what the crowd says or what the circumstances may happen to be.

As you obediently follow Jesus' instructions to pray and keep on praying, God will work. Obedience is your job. The outcome is God's job.

OBEDIENCE REWARDED

Obedience isn't always easy. It's not always comfortable. It doesn't always make sense. It's not always easy to explain. Someone might say to you, "Why pray when no answers have come?" It may sound trite to say, "Well, Jesus says to pray, and I will obey." But that is the key. Jesus said, "Pray." Obediently following Jesus means praying even when we see zero results and zero movement.

Sometimes God gives us a glimpse that our obedience is on track even when the prayers haven't been answered yet. Before moving to Kansas in 2005, our life was pretty good. I was serving in a great church. Lost people were finding Jesus. Great things were happening. The church was growing. The pastoral staff was like family. Everybody was happy. All was good.

Then a guy named Keith Wright, the Church of the Nazarene district superintendent from Kansas City at the time, called me up and said, "Hey, Rob, have I got a church for you . . ." He originally called in September 2004 and I said, "Thanks, but no thanks." Then he called again in January of 2005, and I said we'd come and talk with the church board.

Well, to make a long story short, we believed that Kansas was where God was calling us, and upon the church's invitation we said, "Yes" and became the pastor of the Central Church of the Nazarene. That part of the story you may know (if you read my bio on the back cover of this book). This part you may not know.

On my last night in Michigan, Karla and I had gone to Wal-Mart to pick up some things for the trip. I was going to be leaving the next day to drive to Kansas by myself because we hadn't sold our house yet, and my boys had to finish up the year in their schools. (We didn't want to pull them out of school with six weeks to go in the school year.) So I was packing up Black Betty—my Chevy Impala—and making the final preparation for the trip to Kansas City alone.

The night before leaving, I was in Wal-Mart buying the necessities for the trip: Hot Tamales, Nestle Crunch bars, pretzels, and snacks for the seven-hundred-mile journey from our home in Michigan to Kansas City. As I was going through those aisles of Wal-Mart, it hit me. It really hit me. "I'm really leaving Michigan. This has been my home since birth (with the exception of college and seminary). This is it—I'm buying Hot Tamales for the road, and except for vacations, I'm not coming back to live here."

The next thing that went through my mind was, "What in the world have you done, Rob? You're leaving family and friends. You're leaving a great church—a church that God has blessed in great ways. You're uprooting your family. You don't know anybody in Kansas. What in the world have you done?"

There in the Wal-Mart candy aisle I was having a little crisis.

My mind quickly started calculating:

Maybe I can call the district superintendent and tell him I've changed my mind.

Maybe I can ask the board at Richfield if I can stay.

Maybe they'll give me a mulligan. A do-over. A "Whoops —I was just kidding. I'm not really moving."

All these things were running through my mind. I was praying, "Lord, did I get it right? Do you really want me to move to Kansas City?"

And you are not going to believe this, but right in the middle of my time of doubt and crisis moment, a song came over the Wal-Mart public address system. It was not a Christian song. It wasn't Handel's *Messiah* and the "Hallelujah Chorus"—as if God were saying, "I'm hearing you—Hallelujah! Hallelujah! Hallelujah!" That wasn't the song.

It was better. You're going to think I'm making this up. It's completely true. As I was having my little crisis and asking, "God, what do you want me to do? Have I made a mistake? Should I stay in Michigan? Do you really want me in Kansas City?" over the loud speaker I heard Fats Domino singing his famous song about going to Kansas City.

I couldn't believe it. Of all the songs in the Wal-Mart music repertoire, the song that was playing as I was worried about my move to Kansas City was Fats singing about going to Kansas City? Are you kidding me? I started tearing up. I started crying, right there in Wal-Mart. God turned the Wal-Mart candy aisle into holy ground.

I found Karla and said, "Karla, do you hear what is on the PA system?" She couldn't believe it either. Maybe Fats Domino was on their playlist. Maybe Wal-Mart regularly played that song. Some might say, "What a strange coincidence." All I know is that when I needed to hear a word from the Lord, I heard him, and he sounded a lot like Fats Domino.

God knows what we need and when we need it!

I tell that story to say, walking in obedience while I was at Wal-Mart at that moment was not all that easy. I was having some serious doubts about my decision and the next years of my life. But God came through as if to say: "You're on the right track. You're doing what I want. You're in the right place. Go to Kansas City and chase out the darkness. Storm the gates of hell. You are going where I want you to go."

There was no earth-shattering miracle in Wal-Mart— just Fats Domino reminding me that God was still working and I had nothing to fear.

As we obediently pray, trust, and seek the Lord—even when the specific earth-shattering "Boom! Done! Healed!" miracle doesn't happen, don't be surprised by the little reminders from God that he is still at work and you can trust him.

6 | PAIN AND SIN
THE ROLE OF SINFUL BEHAVIORS AND SICKNESS

Before you read another word in this chapter, read this: your pain may not be the result of sin in your life. I'm not sure I wrote that strong enough, and I'm not sure you read it strong enough, so let me try it again: *your pain may not be the result of sin.* (In fact, it probably isn't.) Still not strong enough—*there is a very good chance that your pain is not the result of sinful behavior.*

But maybe it is.

I hesitated to put this chapter in the book because of all the religious mumbo jumbo concerning the subject of sickness and sin. There has certainly been a lot of bad theology and mounds of guilt heaped upon the innocent victims of tragedy and sickness throughout the centuries. I don't want to add more words to bad theology or unnecessary guilt.

I've seen enough from picket-carrying protesters that equate everything from tornadoes to military members' deaths to a vengeful god. I've heard enough of religious television pundits who offer an explanation for tsunamis and terror attacks as God's judgment upon a sinful nation. I certainly do not want to be counted in their group. I am always a little uneasy (sometimes a lot uneasy) when I hear someone say that "God told me to say . . ." So I will avoid such statements in this discussion.

But I also cannot escape the fact that often in the Bible people saw a direct correlation between sin and sickness. If you were sick or had some sort of ailment, then there was one reason for it: *sin*. It wasn't just the Pharisees or the misinformed that saw it this way.

JOSHUA'S CASE STUDY OF SIN AND TROUBLES

There are a lot of examples in the Old Testament of disobedience leading to sickness or trouble. Just ask Joshua.

The battle for Jericho had been a complete and total success, an overwhelming victory. Joshua had given the battle to the Lord, and the Lord worked in a mighty and impressive fashion. Chapter 6 ends with these words: "So the LORD was with Joshua, and his fame spread throughout the land" (verse 27).

When God's holy and inspired Word says that the Lord is with you and that your fame is spreading throughout the land, that's a pretty good thing. That's better than making *People* magazine's list of the one hundred most beautiful people in the world or *Fortune* magazine's list of the richest people in the world. When the Bible says God is with someone—and if you're that guy that God is with—then you should be on top of the world.

Joshua was the guy! It would be easy to assume that his chest was out. His head held high. No doubt thinking, "All is well! God is with me and my fame is spread throughout the land! Nothing could be finer—even if I were in Carolina—it's good to be me!"

Just on the other side of Jericho was a town called Ai. Twelve thousand folks lived there, as we are told in Joshua 8. It was a Canaanite village. Nothing compared to the big metropolis that Jericho was. There may not have been the huge walls protecting Ai like Jericho. There were no sophisticated warriors like Jericho had. When the spies that Joshua commissioned returned, they reported that there weren't too many men in the town at all. (No doubt they had been on the losing end of a few battles in the past, so the men were gone.) The spies reported that they could defeat Ai with one chariot tied behind their back. Ai would be easy pickings. No problem. A piece of cake.

So Joshua gives the orders. The troops head out to Ai fully expecting another lopsided victory. Probably they were thinking they would all be home in time for lunch, but they quickly discovered that was not going to be the case. Joshua 7:4 plainly states that the men of Israel were "routed" by the men of Ai. These warriors fresh from the heights of victory in Jericho were whipped, beaten, and routed by the teeny, tiny town of Ai. What in the world happened?

I see it all the time. A Christian is doing great—his walk with the Lord is going along just fine. Often God has just done something remarkable in his life. Then another challenge arises (many times not as big as some previous challenge that he has just come through but a smaller challenge), and the believer says, "Humpf . . . I can handle this . . . no problem."

Then, *boom*!

He falls flat on his face and defeat sets in. These folks look around and say exactly what the people of Israel were saying after their battle with Ai: "What in the world happened?"

There are two big reasons for spiritual defeat in the life of a believer: The first I call "super, sensational, superlative self." It's super *me*! The second is from *sin*.

Super, Sensational, Superlative Self

This is the mistaken notion that when you are doing so great and so wonderful and so terrific that you can handle things all on your own. It reminds me of the old story when Muhammad Ali was world champion and was on a plane, and the flight attendant came up to him and said, "Mr. Ali, you will need to fasten your seat belt."

To which he replied, "Superman don't need a seat belt."

The flight attendant's quick reply was: "Superman doesn't need a plane either."

He put on his seatbelt.

We know we are not Superman or Superwoman, but too often we begin to act like it. Such an attitude leads to defeat every time.

It happened to Joshua and the people of Israel. Everything was great, terrific, and wonderful. The walls of Jericho had just come "a tumblin' down." The Lord was with Joshua and his fame was spreading throughout the land—you can't get much better than that—then, *boom!*—defeat.

When times are tough, what do we do? We pray, right? So if you're sick, pray for healing. If the finances are low, pray for help. If our kids are in trouble, we cry out to God on their behalf. If there is a crisis in our job or in our school or in the country—we hit our knees. We have prayer meetings. We get serious.

What happened after 9/11? That next Sunday, the church I pastored was packed. And there were signs all around to "Pray for America." People were praying and seeking God. But what happened after the crisis was over? The prayer meetings ended. Routine set back in. The crisis was over and so was the devotion to God in many people's lives.

It happens all the time—when life gets back to normal, what do we do? When you are feeling fine and the kids are bringing home straight "A's," too often prayer gets sent to the back burner. Someone has suggested that the reason Christians are in trouble so much of the time is that it is the only time the Lord hears from us. Maybe that's true.

Before the battle of Jericho and the battle of Ai, Joshua sent out spies to inspect and check out the land.

Before the battle of Jericho and the battle of Ai, Joshua organized the troops and readied them for battle.

Here is the kicker—before the battle of Jericho, Joshua met with the Lord. But preceding the battle of Ai, nowhere does the Bible indicate that Joshua prayed about the battle. Nowhere does it say that he inquired of the Lord. Nowhere does it say that Joshua met with the Lord or sought God's direction or received God's approval for the battle plans. There was none of that.

I think Joshua (remember: great biblical hero, Joshua—"Strong and Courageous" Joshua; God was with him; his fame was spreading throughout the land—that Joshua) saw this teeny, tiny town of Ai and said, "Oh man, we can handle this. We just defeated Jericho. Ai will be no problem." That's a good indicator that the person has read the press clippings and has bought into the notion that he or she is a "super, sensational, superlative self."

And after the defeat at Ai, Joshua 7:6 tells how Joshua tore his clothes and fell on to the ground and put ashes on his head—all signs of grieving and mourning. And then, he finally cried out to God. Listen to what he says (this is going to surprise you, coming from a great hero of the faith),

Alas, Sovereign LORD, why did you ever bring this people across the Jordan to deliver us into the hands of the Amorites to destroy us? If only we had been content to stay on the other side of the Jordan! Pardon your servant, Lord. What can I say, now that Israel has been routed by its enemies? The Canaanites and the other people of the country will hear about this and they will surround us and wipe out our name from the earth. What then will you do for your own great name? (Joshua 7:7-9)

Does that sound like a hero's prayer? "Why did you bring us out to have us destroyed? O Lord, what can I say to you? Boo hoo." Does that sound like the same strong leader who in chapter 1 said, "Be strong and courageous . . . for the LORD will be with you wherever you go?" (verse 9). Is this the same guy who the Bible says, "The Lord was with Joshua, and his fame spread throughout the land" (6:27)? Yup. It's the same guy.

The portrait of the spiritually defeated is not very pretty, is it? And it doesn't take long to go from the mountaintop to the valley. Despite how high Joshua was when "his fame was spreading throughout the land," now he is in the pit of despair.

Let me just state that if Joshua—a hero of the faith for sure; a guy known far and wide; a man who encouraged others to be strong and courageous; a man who went against the prevailing opinion and was faithful to God—if he can get defeated and struggle, then guess what? I've got news for you—it could happen to you and me. We are not exempt.

So Joshua is defeated and you get the feeling that the Lord gets a wee bit tired of it. Do you see what God said in Joshua 7:10-12? "Stand up! What are you doing down on your face? Israel has sinned; they have violated my covenant, which I commanded them to keep. They have taken some of the devoted things; they have stolen, they have lied, they have put them with their own possessions. That is why the Israelites cannot stand against their enemies."

In other words, God is saying, "Sin is the problem. Plain and simple. Sin is the problem."

Spiritual defeat can come from our "super, sensational, superlative self," but spiritual defeat can also come from *sin*.

Sin

Sin is a direct path to destruction. I'm not saying that every defeat is a result of sin, but I am saying that every sin leads to defeat. Do you see the difference?

For our discussion, not every pain is the result of sin, but it is entirely possible that some of our sickness is the result of sin.

Let's get one thing straight. God hates sin. He always has; he always will. God will not honor sinful behavior. God loves everybody, but he does not bless everyone. If you are involved in sinful activity, if you are doing things that you know God is not happy with, then you are not pleasing God. God gives us the freedom to make poor choices, but do not expect his blessing while you are making those sinful choices. If you are sinning in one area of your life, then don't expect God to bless you in another area of your life. It's not going to happen.

SIN ALWAYS LEADS TO DEFEAT—ALWAYS

In Israel's case, even though God plainly told the people not to take any of the spoils of the battle, Achan, a soldier in Israel's army, did just that. He swiped a little bit of gold, a little bit of silver, and a fancy Babylonian robe.

Now I can't say for certain what was going through Achan's brain when the battle of Jericho was going on. I seriously doubt that he thought about disobeying God before the walls of Jericho came a tumblin' down. I doubt that this was a premeditated act. My guess is that in the midst of the confusion of battle, Achan came across the loot and rather than turning it in as required, he kept it for himself. It was a spontaneous thing. Sin can happen so quickly. Let your guard down even for a moment and your vulnerabilities and weakness will be exposed. It happened to Achan.

No doubt he rationalized his sin: "No one will miss a little gold and a little silver. What's God going to do with this fancy Babylonian robe? It's not like he's going to be wearing it at a heavenly banquet. It's no big deal. Who will even notice? What will it hurt?"

How wrong Achan was!

Your sin always affects more than you. It affects your thinking. It affects who you are and the way you approach life. It affects the people you know and the people you love. Your sin affects your family. Your friends. Your church. It affects your well-being both emotionally and physically. Sin messes up every relationship, every thought pattern, and every hope and dream.

I have heard the argument that God dealt differently with the people in the Old Testament than he does after Jesus and the New Testament. I believe it is true. Achan was living in an era different from us. I get it that the primitive people in Israel's infancy learned through a system of rewards and punishments. So God would approach them with the conditional statements like, "If you obey, you will be blessed." I get it that God wants our obedience not because it is beneficial to us or because of what we will "get out of it" but because it is right. I get all of that.

GOD REALLY HATES SIN

I am not sure if we even come close to understanding just how much God hates sin. He really hates it. Paul warns the believers in Corinth the consequences of not honoring God in the way they participate in Communion by saying, "That is why many of you are weak and sick and some have even died" (1 Corinthians 11:30, NLT). When James discussed the power of healing, he indicated that a prerequisite to healing is confessing our sins to each other. It sure seems that sin—as Paul and James understood it—doesn't affect us just spiritually but physically as well.

Possibly because of our zeal to talk about an all-loving, all-forgiving God, we push to the back of our mind a God who allows the consequences of sin to impact a person's life. It's not a popular position to say that God allows sickness. But does he?

Is it out of the realm of possibility to think that if a person is participating in behaviors that they absolutely know are not pleasing God that God would allow that person to endure pain or a physical setback to remind them of their need for him and/or their need to confess? I really don't think that is such a crazy notion.

If much pain is the result of stress, is it really a stretch to think that a person living in open rebellion against God would be filled with stress and in turn have some physical consequences as a result of that stress and sin?

Make sure you understand my position. I am not suggesting the God sends pain as punishment. I am suggesting that God allows pain as a result of sinful behavior. That's true if the pain is the result of binge drinking the night before or if the pain is the result of stress from rebelling against a holy God.

If someone is participating in sinful behaviors while at the same time experiencing pain, should God be obligated (God is God; is he ever "obligated" to us? I don't think so—but for the sake of argument, should God be obligated) to answer a prayer for healing? Again, is God required to respond positively to a prayer for healing when the person is living his or her life in a manner that is contrary to God? I think it is much more likely, God would say, "You are choosing your path. Walk in it. Get back to me when you decide it's time to start following me with all of your life."

CONFESSION AND HEALING

James's advice for those seeking healing seems to be pretty good counsel. The old proverb says, "Confession is good for the soul"—maybe it's good for the body as well.

Again, I am not saying every pain (or even most pain) is the result of sin. I am saying that some pain very possibly could be the result of sinfulness. So the first step in healing should be an open and honest conversation with the Lord. Take an inventory of your behaviors and attitudes. Are there any hindrances in your relationship with him? Is there anything standing between you and a holy God? Are there areas of your life that are not pleasing to him?

Do you have grudges or bitterness harbored against someone in your life? Is there someone you need to forgive? Jesus instructed during the Sermon on the Mount: "If you are offering your gift at the altar and there remember that your brother or sister has something against you, leave your gift there in front of the altar. First go and be reconciled to them; then come and offer your gift" (Matthew 5:23-24). It makes sense that our requests for pain relief should be in a similar order. Are we asking God to bring us healing while at the same time we have been refusing to be a source of healing with a brother or sister?

I write this not to add another ache to the chronic pain sufferer. Healthy periodical soul examinations are good for us. Like David's response, a good prayer is still, "Search me, God, and know my heart; test me and know my anxious thoughts. See if there is any offensive way in me, and lead me in the way everlasting" (Psalm 139:23-24).

Some pain might be the result of sin. Some healing may be prevented because of sin or harbored bad feelings toward another person. Maybe the most proactive pain "treatment" is to examine your relationship with God and with others. If such an examination results in confession and reconciliation, then even if the pain is not immediately removed, you are still better off than you were. Pain relief begins with a clear conscience and a confessing heart.

OUR COMMON PRACTICE: CONFESSION

James wrote, "Make this your common practice: Confess your sins to each other and pray for each other so that you can live together whole and healed" (James 5:16, TM). For James, confession was an acceptable, needed act that leads to wholeness and healing. It was to be a "common" practice.

A "common practice" is something that happens a lot. Brushing my teeth is a common practice that I do two or three times a day. Eating is a common practice that I do three times a day. Corporate worship is a common practice that happens at least once a week. When was the last time you confessed anything to anybody? Could you really refer to your confessional behavior as a "common practice"?

At the church I pastor, one Sunday we talked about confession and at the end of the teaching time, rather than a traditional altar call, we provided confessional cards to everyone in the sanctuary. I asked people to confess attitudes and/or behaviors that were less than pleasing to God. I called on people to admit to those things that were keeping them from having "the mind of Christ."

The response was overwhelming.

Hundreds of people moved forward and dropped their confessional card into one of two boxes. One box was labeled "junk" (I promised that no one would read the cards dropped in the "junk" box, and I have no idea how many cards were placed in it), and the other box was labeled "shared junk" where I would read and pray for the people and the troubling areas of their life. In the "shared junk" box there were 195 cards.

That next week I read and prayed over all 195 cards from the "shared junk" box. Some people confessed to selfishness, anger, worry, or greed. Others confessed fears and various sins. Nineteen confessed to an addiction to pornography. There was a lot of junk in that box. The truth is, we all have junk. Some of us have more junk than others, but we all have junk. The way to move beyond our junk, according to James, is to make confession our common practice.

Moreover, know this: *God's grace is bigger than all of our junk*. There is no sin, worry, problem, or fear that God cannot handle. Confession is the first step to freedom. In fact the Bible says: "If we confess our sins to him, he is faithful and just to forgive us our sins and to cleanse us from all wickedness" (1 John 1:9, NLT). You need not be gripped in the debilitating grasp of sin—God's grace is greater! He is able to cleanse all that junk and all the guilt and give you the mind of Christ!

Confession is a big part in God's transformative work in our lives. It is the place where true healing begins. Chronic pain might not be your biggest trouble. Unconfessed sin may be the stressor that is standing between you and God's perfect peace for your life. Healing and help are found in the humbled heart of a contrite follower of Christ.

Sin may not be the cause of your pain. But pain can be the result of sin and the stress that sin brings into a person's life. Confession and turning from all things contrary to God is the beginning of the healing process in your life—whether or not you suffer from pain.

7 PAIN AND LIFE
DOING ALL THAT YOU CAN DO

I once heard someone say, "Work like everything depends on you; pray like everything depends on God." I think that philosophy is crucial for those of us that deal with chronic pain (as long as you remember that everything really depends on God).

I think the praying like everything depends on God part is easy. When I have an especially bad headache—an eleven on a scale of one to ten—I am a praying machine. I pray like there's no tomorrow. I pray, pray, pray. Praying isn't the issue.

But the working like everything depends on me part is sometimes easy to forget. It's easy to get lazy. It's easy to just pray and say "I have faith that God will heal me," then sit around, patiently waiting for God to heal, and do nothing in the meantime to help the situation. Maybe a pastor isn't supposed to say this, but sometimes we need to get up and do something.

In other words, I need to do all that I can do to get well. In the last chapter, the point was that we need to make sure that sin or a poor relationship with others is not hindering the work of God in our life. But there are other things besides a spiritual evaluation that we can do, such as:

Eat well.

Sleep well.

Exercise.

Listen to your doctors.

Have a healthy mind-set and a healthy attitude.

EATING RIGHT

In my case, my doctor is convinced that proper nutrition plays a role in headaches. In fact, he said the second most important book to the Bible is David Buchholz's *Heal Your Headache: The 1-2-3 Program for Taking Charge of Your Pain.* My doctor convinced me that there are plenty of "headache triggers" in various foods that we eat. So, on one awful day a few years ago now, I was sitting in his office and we were discussing my headache issues and he instructed me in no uncertain terms that I needed to take seriously the migraine diet he advocated.

What kind of diet, you ask? Why did I refer to it as an "awful" day? Imagine every food that tastes good (got them pictured in your brain?); now imagine all those tasty items being on the "no-no" list. Well, it is not quite that bad, but it is close. There are some good foods I can eat, but they will have to be prepared in such a bland and tasteless manner that even my dog would prefer her Purina. The list includes no dairy, no sauces, no soups, no chocolate, no caffeine, no citrus, no Chinese, no bananas, no raspberries, no nuts, no alcohol, no tobacco, no onions (do you know how many foods contain onions? a lot!), no tomatoes, some other veggies, no fresh baked things (of course thanks to also needing to have a gluten-free diet most yummy baked items were already off the list), no processed meats, no fish, no salty snacks, no MSG . . . no kidding.

I've got to be honest with you—I like food. I don't like food like the *Bizarre Food* guy on the Travel Channel likes food. I wouldn't like eating some weird rodent from a foreign country. And I don't like food like the *Man vs. Food* guy likes food. I'm not advocating gluttony. But I sure do like a perfectly seasoned steak grilled medium well, with a fully loaded baked potato and a tasty side of baked beans. (My mouth is watering just thinking about it.) I like Chinese food, Mexican food, Italian food, and barbecue. I like it spicy. I like it with friends. I like it under candlelight with just Karla and me. Food is good.

But my doctor told me, "Food is fuel." He gave a convincing argument that its purpose is for nothing more than to keep the body working. Obviously, he never tasted Myrtle Weber's meatloaf at a church potluck!

Looking over the list of possible triggers gave me a sick feeling in my stomach. I knew what it meant. To abide by the diet would take discipline and would eliminate many of my favorite foods. It would leave me as one of those people who are food kooky. Food kooky people ask a lot of questions at restaurants and are extremely picky at potlucks. Food kooky people can easily be mistaken for a food snobby person, and that is even worse. A food snobby person behaves as if his or her food is better than all other entrées prepared by even the finest chefs. I did not want to be a food kooky or a food snobby person.

I also did not want to have headaches. There came a point where attempting to find pain relief trumped my fear of being labeled a food freak.

So long, Mexican food.

Good-bye, hot dogs.

Ciao, chili.

Taking charge of your pain means doing what you can as it relates to your diet.

It seems silly to pray for God to heal you and take away the pain, while at the same time doing little to help your situation or even negatively contributing to your situation. Like praying grace before a meal of an extra-large, greasy fast-food burger and extra-salty fries and super-sized sugary soda and then asking God to "make the meal nourishment to your body." Jesus turned water into wine; he did not turn a double beef, extra-cheese grease burger into a salad with low-fat dressing. Doing what you can means taking your diet seriously.

PROPER EXERCISE

I will admit I hate exercise. Some people love it. Live for it. Can't wait to do it. It's the highlight of their day. That's not me. I hate it with a deep, bitter hatred. For years, I thought I didn't have time. I could not devote the necessary time to exercise on a consistent basis. I lied to myself that I was in reasonable shape. How could exercise help my pain?

Of course, every doctor I've been to has asked me how much I was exercising. They have all said exercise is good for heart health but also good for head health. Every doctor with anything more than a Cracker Jack medical degree will say, "More exercise, less weight, more sleep, less alcohol and to-bacco, and less stress are the key factors in headache control."

Exercise began for me just as taking control of my diet did. One day I woke up and said, "I've got to take this seriously." I started running. Not far at first. But each time I ran (three or four times a week) I determined to run a little bit farther than I had run the previous day until I reached my desired time and distance. I adjusted my schedule and would not give in to the temptation to not exercise. I knew if I was going to develop a habit of exercise it would mean doing it when I didn't feel like it. Running even with a headache (when you have a headache five out of seven days and you are also trying to run four out of seven days, then obviously many of those runs will be occurring with a headache), I was determined that I would not stop exercising.

Okay . . . I started to eat right. Then I started exercising more. Next question—how do I manage my stress?

MANAGING STRESS

Stress is a contributing factor in headaches for me. (In a later chapter I will address the unique issues of pastoring and pain control.) I have already mentioned that my brain hemorrhage occurred during a particularly stressful time in my life. It should not be a news flash to recognize that good stress management will coincide with pain management.

Honesty alert: I do not have this figured out. I'm working on it. I know the verses I need to know in regard to this. Verses like: "Do not be anxious about anything, but in every situation, by prayer and petition, with thanksgiving, present your requests to God. And the peace of God, which transcends all understanding, will guard your hearts and your minds in Christ Jesus" (Philippians 4:6-7). Or Jesus' simple words in the Sermon on the Mount: "Do not worry about your life" (Matthew 6:25). Those are just a couple of the verses that tell us to leave our troubles and stress with Jesus.

I also know how difficult it is to actually leave our stress with him. My doctors said my blood pressure spiked on the day of my brain hemorrhage. Prior to that day, I had never had an issue with high blood pressure. I also wasn't eating properly. My diet was a mess. I was unaware of a gluten intolerance issue. I wasn't exercising. My sleep was a disaster. There were more stressful issues than at any point in my ministry (by far). You don't have to have a medical degree from Harvard to say that was a recipe for disaster. I was letting the stress win. It had gotten the better of me, and I was ill-prepared to handle it.

Here's what I've been discovering—the more I take care of the things I can take care of (diet, exercise, sleep, and taking periodical spiritual inventories to make sure everything between God and me is up-to-date) the easier it is to manage my stress. If I am eating right, getting enough sleep, exercising, and at peace with God, I seem to be better equipped to handle the stressful moments of life and ministry. Stress comes into all of our lives, but it does not have to overcome us.

DON'T LET THE PAIN WIN

Even after the brain hemorrhage recovery and as the headaches have continued, I have had to make lifestyle decisions about sleep, exercise, and diet. I have also decided to not let the pain win.

I've always been a tad competitive, and I started to take a competitive approach to my migraines. I decided I was not going to let the pain win. Pain wins if it completely ruins everything about your day. Pain wins when you become so agitated that no one wants to be around you. Pain wins if you are so inward focused that you don't see or care about what is going on around you. Pain wins when everything productive stops and nothing good is happening.

Conversely, the pain does not win when even though it's throbbing, your kids know that you love them. So for example, when you are in a dark, noiseless room and your child or grandchild happens by the room, winning a battle over the pain means calling the child over and giving her a hug. You could offer a kiss on the forehead. It's reminding her that her hugs and kisses always make you feel a little bit better. Will the hug wipe out the pain? Probably not. But that headache will win the day in that child's mind or yours if you allow moments of love and normality to pass by. Knowing you can still connect with your loved ones even as the excruciating pain rages will bring a certain amount of satisfaction in spite of the situation.

There are times when one must realize, "I'm going to be in pain if I am in bed cut off from the world, and I'm going to be in pain if I am with the family." So given a choice (and sometimes the pain is so incredibly bad there is no choice, but when you have a choice) choose to not let the pain win and join the family activity. Of course, if the particular activity creates a pain-inducing situation, you may want to avoid it. Will you enjoy the activity as much as if you didn't have pain? Who are we kidding? No. It is not easy to be at a function with pain. But at the end of the day, the pain didn't win. Your family is worth sucking it up and toughing it out every now and then.

I recently visited my mom for a few days, and I also had tickets to a University of Michigan football game. Funny how those two events happened together. . . . Anyway, the game day arrived. It was a beautiful autumn afternoon. Absolutely gorgeous. It was a perfect day to be with my closest 110,000 friends in Ann Arbor. I also had a raging headache. I could have called the friend I was going to the game with and say, "Listen, this headache is killing me, and I can't go." Or I could refuse to let the headache win. I could take some medicine and hope that the headache would rage a little less (not an easy task when the greatest marching band in the world is in the house—even if it's a "Big House," the band is still loud). I went to the game. Did the headache go away? No, but I think it was helped by a sixty-three to thirteen Wolverine victory. And the headache didn't win the day. That's my point.

DAVID'S FIGHTING WORDS

Before David gave Goliath the headache of his life, do you remember how he advocated his capabilities to King Saul to fight the giant? He said, "The LORD who rescued me from the paw of the lion and the paw of the bear will rescue me from the hand of this Philistine" (1 Samuel 17:37). In other words, God was with me in the past against pretty formidable foes, and God will be with me in this fight against a bigger foe. Someone once said, "King Saul and the Israelites saw Goliath and said he was too big to kill. David saw Goliath and thought he was too big to miss." I love it!

In the same vein, I can say, "The Lord who rescued me from the pain of a migraine so massive it was like someone was hitting me with a Louisville Slugger will rescue me from this headache too." The bigger the headache, the bigger my desire to see God work in great ways in my life! When a massive migraine is booming, I remind my nasty headache that my God is bigger than any headache known to man. I need not fear. I need not worry. Headaches are no challenge to the God of the universe.

FIGHTING THE FIGHT WITH GOD

Fighting has never been my forte. When you are the smallest kid in your class from kindergarten to graduation, you learn pretty quickly that fighting might not be in your best interest. Knowing my size, my folks told me if I ever was confronted by a bigger, stronger kid (read: every boy and most of the girls in my school), then I needed to do a lot of "cutting and shooting"—cutting around corners and shooting for home. I took their advice all but one time. That lone exception was not pretty. A pay-per-view classic it would not have been.

It was in seventh grade math class. A rather large boy named John took exception to some comments I had made about his intelligence or lack thereof and decided to hit me. (Looking back years later, I now see that John's intelligence should never have been questioned, but mine, on the other hand, maybe should have been. John was twice my size and twice as mean.) So what I lacked in muscles, size, and speed, I made up for with an equal lack of tact and discernment. Anyway, I mouthed off to John and he hit me. He didn't slap me. He hit me. Hard. If it were an old Batman episode, the TV screen would have displayed a big "POW!" There were actually two hits in this fight. John hit me and I hit the ground. End of fight. End of story. This was no David vs. Goliath remake. I had no time to say, "John, you come against me with big muscles and strong fists, but I come against you in the name of the Lord Almighty." I didn't say that. I didn't have time to run down to the babbling brook and grab five smooth stones for my slingshot. (I didn't even own a slingshot, and the only thing babbling at Radcliff Junior High was me, not a brook.)

The truth is that my giant battle could have been avoided if I had simply kept quiet and played nice. Not all battles are that way. Not all giants are like John. Sometimes we are confronted with giants—maybe not with big fists like John or with swords and shields like Goliath—but giants nonetheless. There are plenty of giants lurking these days that will not go away by playing nice and keeping quiet. I've known plenty of people battling the giant of drug addiction or the giant of depression. There are giants of selfishness, pornography, and alcoholism. And the topic of this book, the giant of pain and suffering, can be very formidable.

When confronting these modern-day giants, grabbing a couple of stones from the closest brook won't help, but grabbing hold of God surely will. Like David, we need to proclaim that our God is able to deliver us and help us move forward with courage and faith. It's a matter of trusting that God will do what's best and obediently following him.

Doing what you can in the headache battle is being an active participant in the fight. Could God have sent a lightning bolt and struck down Goliath, thereby sparing David of the slingshot duel of all time (and severely limiting the pregame speeches of underdog sports teams for all time)? Of course! Instead, God chose to use a willing, faithful participant named David to get the job done. In your battle, don't sit on the sidelines waiting for God to work a miracle. Become an active participant in your treatment, doing all you can to defeat this foe. Whether or not God heals you (in this life) is out of your control, but doing what you can in the midst of your pain is totally in your control.

8 PAIN AND THE CALENDAR
WAITING WITHOUT RELIEF

Prior to my brain hemorrhage, I hadn't spent a lot of time in doctors' office waiting rooms. I've been to plenty of hospitals and have spent time in many surgical waiting rooms with families while a loved one is undergoing a surgical procedure. But I had not visited too many doctors' office waiting rooms. There is a difference between the two waiting rooms. Surgical waiting rooms are sometimes tense when the family is uncertain of the outcome in the operating room, but usually they are a little boring. Everyone is trying to pass the time. The people in a surgical waiting room aren't sick. They are bored or worried or both—but most generally they are healthy.

It's different in a doctor's office waiting room. There are sick folks in there. I remember when I had my first checkup with my neurosurgeon. He had a nice office with nice, comfortable chairs in the waiting room. The night before, the janitorial crew had done a good job. The room was clean and smelled nice. But as I sat in the room waiting for my name to be called, I looked at all the other patients that were waiting to see the doctor too. Silly admission alert—I'm not an Olympic athlete. Still, I was easily the healthiest-looking person in the room. Because I didn't actually need brain surgery and since I had no visible side effects from the hemorrhage, I was different from the other patients in the room. All the others showed visible signs of a stroke or brain injury of some kind. There were a lot of troubled people in that room.

The office is in America, with all the advances of modern medicine. Still, that waiting room was not a happy place. Suffering and troubled people were in every corner of the room. No one was joking or playing games. They were all waiting to see a doctor and hoping for relief.

A LONG, LONG WAIT

Now try to imagine the suffering people waiting for a miracle at Bethesda in the first century. Bethesda is the location of a great healing in John 5. John tells us that Bethesda was the name of a pool by the Sheep Gate in Jerusalem. But don't think of this place as a resort spa in some exotic location, or even like your neighborhood pool with wild, squirt-gun-wielding second graders running around. It was more like my neurosurgeon's waiting room—only without the comfy chairs and pleasant aroma.

There were a lot of troubled people there. John says it had "a great number of disabled people" there. The blind, lame, and paralyzed people would hang out, hoping for a miracle or a few coins tossed into their hat from those passing by the area. How many people make up a "great number"? I'm not sure, but think of your busiest inner-city hospital emergency room and multiply the horror by a thousand and you still wouldn't be close to the scene at Bethesda. One of those in the "great number" of suffering souls was a man who had been an invalid for thirty-eight years. Thirty-eight years! That's a long time. If you have been doing something or being somewhere for thirty-eight years (no matter what it is), that's a long time.

Imagine how this guy felt—an invalid for thirty-eight years. Year in and year out, day in and day out, waking to the same reality that he could not walk and was at the mercy of those who might toss him a few coins as he begged for his very survival. The difficulty, the awful reality of his life, is nearly incomprehensible to we who are living in the United States in the twenty-first century. Like being a widow in the first century, being physically handicapped in the first century would not be easy. There were no ramps for the handicapped, no wheelchairs, no prescription medications, no BENGAY, no heating pads, no meals on wheels, no social security, and no Medicaid. There was no help for a person in his situation. It was a pitiful existence for thirty-eight long, terrible, horrible, miserable years.

Another thing you need to remember—twenty centuries ago in Jerusalem, the average life span was somewhere south of forty years. Do the math—this guy had been in this condition for a lifetime.

Then he met Jesus!

There are other biblical figures who also struggled for years with their particular issue. The man from John 9 was born blind. I don't know how old he was, but he was old enough to be on his own and speak for himself (according to his parents). He was considered an adult. And then there was the lady who had a bleeding disorder for twelve years until she touched Jesus' cloak. In the Old Testament, Abraham and Sarah were told they were going to have a baby but then had to wait years and years before hearing the pitter-patter of little feet in their bungalow. And Moses was on the "far side of the desert" for forty years before he encountered God at the burning bush. All of those heroes no doubt had been praying for God's miraculous working in their lives, and they all had to wait a long, long time before anything happened.

Most of us have a hard time suffering for a season. But a lot of folks in the Bible did just that.

THE TROUBLE WITH WAITING

We have a hard time waiting even a little bit. Sadly, I admit to getting annoyed standing in the express lane at Wal-Mart for more than five minutes. If our fast food is not fast enough, we get annoyed. At times, believers have been known to take that same approach with God. We sometimes think, "Hey, I prayed. I've waited. I've placed my order (as if we can order God). Where's the service? (As if God is required to serve us.) It's been a few days or even a few weeks—why hasn't God answered my prayers?" Maybe one result of our lifestyles with express checkout lanes, instant messaging, and rapid response is that we think everything should happen right now. God included.

Too often, we think "long term" is days or weeks. But could it be we need to think in years? (Not that I want to have these noggin thumpers for years, mind you.) It's hard to imagine it has been five years since my brain hemorrhage. That seems like a long time, on the one hand, but like the time has flown by on the other. I am sure that I am learning a lot during this period in my life. And while I do not have it all figured out (not by a long shot), I know this for sure: I can trust God's timing, whether healing comes in days, months, years, or heaven.

The people in the church I pastor are probably tired of me saying this, but it's true: God is rarely early. He is never late. He is always right on time. And just for the record, I know God is far more concerned about who I am becoming in this journey than how quickly I arrive at some destination.

Maybe the key to relief is to quit praying for a rescue and start praying for revelation. Throughout eternity we will not be focused on our pain; instead, we will be thankful for who we became in Christ through the painful times. Sometimes the glorious work of God happens when we think nothing is happening.

WAITING WITH UNANSWERED PRAYERS

I am guessing during the thirty-eight-year wait, the crippled man at Bethesda had plenty of time to wonder why God hadn't answered his prayers. I don't know whether or not he came up with a list of reasons, but here's my list of why prayers can go unanswered.

1. **It's a dumb prayer.** Now, I don't think praying for pain relief is a dumb prayer. And I don't think the guy who had been disabled for thirty-eight years was praying dumb prayers. But I've heard plenty of people pray for dumb things. God doesn't answer dumb prayers. Dumb prayers include prayers that contradict other prayers or prayers that are detrimental to others. Dumb prayers are prayers that are demanding. Dumb prayers assume that God is at the mercy of our whims and desires. Dumb prayers sound a lot like a spoiled child's wish list. God doesn't answer dumb prayers.

2. **The person who prays has sin or disobedience in his or her life.** (See the previous chapter.) The short answer to this type of prayer is: Why would God give an affirmation to a prayer when the requester has repeatedly turned his or her back on God's desires? Don't expect a yes from God when your actions repeatedly say no to him.

3. **The person who prays does not have a reconciling attitude.** (See the previous chapter.) If a person can't

make even the most modest attempt to reconcile with family members or people he or she has hurt, then why would God reward the lack of concern for others with a miraculous intervention?

4. **The person who prays has selfish motivations**. I suppose one could make the argument that self-motivated prayers are also dumb prayers. I would agree, but they are so frequently prayed that they need to have their own category. Again, praying for relief from a headache is not usually selfishly motivated unless there is some self-centered agenda behind the request. Praying, "God, heal me of this pain so that I can make a billion dollars or obtain fame and glory for myself" could be labeled a selfishly motivated type of prayer.

5. **God has something better for us**. This one is tough when battling pain. The idea that God could have something better than pain relief is hard to swallow. But as I've discussed about my case, there have been many benefits from my headaches. While I hate to admit that I wasn't an effective pastor before the brain hemorrhage, God has used my headaches to make me a better pastor and person. Could I have become this way without the pain? I'd like to think so, but I don't know.

6. **We discover that God is better than what we are praying for.** This is similar to God having something better for us, only in this case it is God himself who is better for us. If we draw closer to God than ever before, in the scope of eternity, wouldn't that be better than momentary pain relief? Paul described his long list of troubling times and the way he viewed them this way:

> Therefore we do not lose heart. Though outwardly we are wasting away, yet inwardly we are being renewed day by day. For our light and momentary

troubles are achieving for us an eternal glory that far outweighs them all. So we fix our eyes not on what is seen, but on what is unseen, since what is seen is temporary, but what is unseen is eternal. (2 Corinthians 4:16-18)

We are going to spend a whole lot more time in eternity than on earth with these "light and momentary" trials. So doesn't it make sense that if it takes pain (or any other suffering) to draw us nearer to the heart of God, our attitude might be, "Bring it on!" It's all about fixing our eyes on the unseen Eternal One.

7. **God's timing is better than our timing.** This seems to be the case in the man born blind in John 9. Jesus explained that "this happened so that the works of God might be displayed in him" (verse 3). The healing happened in God's timing. God's plan and will would be accomplished on that day in this man's life. When is the optimal time for a healing? I have my ideas, but God's idea is always better than mine.

When suffering with pain, *wait* is a word that no one I know wants to hear. We would much prefer, "Boom! Done!" The character of real faith is seen when we respond similarly whether the word we hear from the Lord is *wait* or *done.*

9 | PAIN AND LONGING FOR HEAVEN
WHEN LIFE SEEMS UNBEARABLE

I've been longing for heaven a little bit today. A place where there will be . . .

No headaches.

No dark rooms.

No worry about loud noises.

No medications.

No Botox.

No shots.

No vitamins.

No migraine diets.

No hospitals, clinics, or doctors' offices.

No blood pressure cuffs.

No thermometers.

No cold stethoscopes.

No MRIs or CT scans.

No physical therapy.

No IVs.

No sleepless nights.

No bifocals, c-pap machines, or oxygen tanks.

No ibuprofen, Tylenol, or BENGAY.

No grieving.

No pain.

No sickness.

But also . . .

No hurt feelings.

No little white lies. No big black lies. No lies period.

No abuse.

No hidden agendas.

No secrets.

No accidents.

No computer problems.

No phone calls from couples telling me they are splitting up.

No brokenhearted teenagers crying tears about not fitting in.

No complaints that the music is too soft, too loud, too old, or too new.

No one picking up and moving to a different mansion on the other side of heaven.

No troubled parents.

No cancer reports.

No dentists' drills.

No biting chiggers or mosquitoes or spiders.

No leaky mansion roofs or basements.

No allergies.

No bad drivers.

None of those things.

And of course, best of all—drumroll please—Jesus! There will be Jesus.

Listen, I know we need to live in the here and now and not be so "heavenly minded that we're no earthly good." I get all that. It's just that there are days when I'm longing for my heavenly home just a little bit.

There are days when it is so easy to get frustrated with migraines that the notion of a place without that brain-busting struggle and worry sounds so incredibly good.

Besides the pain, there are times when I get so tired of tasting my sneakers because I've put my foot in my mouth, or tired of overreacting toward someone I care for and then knowing I need to apologize. I get tired of seeing news reports of war and terrorism, sickness, trouble, abuse, and heartache. I just get tired of our sinful world.

GROANING FOR OUR HEAVENLY DWELLING

I can relate to Paul's heart longings when he wrote in a letter to the Corinthians: "Meanwhile we groan, longing to be clothed instead with our heavenly dwelling" (2 Corinthians 5:2).

That's when I like to read in the Bible that there is coming a day when we followers of Jesus will be in heaven and the worries, cares, and trouble of this old world will be no more. That sounds good to me! It motivates me to tell everybody of this wonderful place that God is preparing for his own. It encourages me to keep my eye on the prize and to keep pressing on. Oh, I can't wait! It's no wonder we used to sing, "When we all get to heaven, what a day of rejoicing that will be!"

It's a natural reaction to our earthly sufferings to want to move on to the "day of rejoicing." It's easy to long for a better place with no sufferings, no worries, and no pain.

When my migraines were at their worst, day after day with no relief, I thought, "Lord, I'm ready to go to heaven." I wasn't suicidal. I was just so ready for a day when there would be no sickness or pain. I was ready for my headache to be over. I was ready to put an end to the suffering. But I wasn't really ready for heaven. And neither was my family ready for me to go to heaven. I was ready for the migraine to be done—for all of my migraines to be over.

LIVING FAR BEYOND OUR ABILITY TO ENDURE

Paul's second letter to the Corinthians has helped me so much through the darkest of days, as he told the group of believers of his life situation. He wrote:

We do not want you to be uninformed, brothers and sisters, about the troubles we experienced in the province of Asia. We were under great pressure, far beyond our ability to endure, so that we despaired of life itself. Indeed, we felt we had received the sentence of death. But this happened that we might not rely on ourselves but on God, who raises the dead. He has delivered us from such a deadly peril, and he will deliver us again. On him we have set our hope that he will continue to deliver us. (2 Corinthians 1:8-10)

I think Paul hit very close to where I was living in saying the pressure upon his life was "far beyond" his ability to endure. Not just "beyond" his ability to endure, but "far beyond." I've been there, Paul! Being under pressure far beyond our ability to endure is a place I was living for several months in the worst moments. Paul testified that he relied on God and God's faithfulness to deliver him in the past. He trusted God's promise of deliverance in the future. I knew that is where I needed to be too. I knew that my only hope was in Christ.

When struggling and suffering, it is so easy to slip into thinking that our troubles are the only problems in the world. Or that God has not and will not come through for us. That's why I need the reminder from Paul every now and then. It puts life with headaches in perspective.

I am not exactly sure where Paul was when writing this second letter to the Corinthians. Probably he was somewhere in Macedonia. I can't speculate on his living conditions or who was with him, although he mentions that Timothy was there. This is what I do know—the type of faulty thinking that leads to a self-focused and destructive place is usually a place of isolation and loneliness.

For me, the progression of self-focus and an unhealthy mind-set happened like this. My head was pounding—really pounding. This was the summer before I began Botox treatments and during the time that I would go into the doctor's office twice a week to be hooked up to an IV drip in an attempt to alleviate the pain with a concoction of medicines. It rarely worked and made me extremely sleepy. Once the medicine was in me, I would go home and climb in bed where I would stay for the rest of the night. This happened week after week.

The IV treatments were not working. Not really. The migraine would briefly subside, but it would always be back the next day, sometimes worse than before the treatment. I was in constant pain.

I spent a lot of time in a dark and quiet place every day. Retreating to my bedroom while the rest of the family was outside on the beautiful Kansas summer nights became a very lonely place. They would have cookouts or swim parties and have friends over, and I was in my bed, pillow over my head, praying and hoping that the headache nightmare would be over.

It didn't take long to start feeling sorry for myself, longing for heaven, and questioning whether or not God would deliver. I was in the "beyond my ability to endure" point. But I still hadn't gotten to my "far beyond" spot. That would come after I thought I had received my answer to my relief and troubles.

My doctor suggested Botox treatments. This was before the FDA had approved Botox for the treatment of headaches. He had been treating people with Botox for some time for individuals who would pay for the treatment out of pocket. (I doubt any of those patients were living on a preacher's salary.) He said, "The IVs aren't working. The medications aren't working. Our next shot (no pun intended) is Botox. I am going to submit your case to your insurance company." But then he added, "Don't get your hopes up. The last twenty-five submissions that I have made to an insurance company for Botox have been rejected."

I started to pray. So did many others on my behalf. And it was just a few days later that the receptionist called me with the good news. The insurance company had agreed that Botox was the best option for me. Twenty-five straight rejections did not intimidate God.

I think in my excitement for this new treatment, I didn't ask a lot of questions. My attitude was, "Let's just get this done!"

One of the questions I didn't ask was, "How long before the Botox effects kick in?" I assumed that it would be immediate. I thought I would walk in with the booming headache that I had been carrying around with me for the last four months, receive the thirty-five or forty shots in my dome, and walk out a new man. Boom! Healed! Done! Instant relief is what I expected to happen. I thought I would be walking out of the clinic as a transformed, migraine-free, ready-to-storm-the-gates-of-hell preacher because I wasn't dealing with headaches any longer. My miracle was about to happen. I was so excited.

That's not what happened.

Somewhere during that treatment the doctor informed me (he may have said it earlier and in my excitement I just didn't hear it) that it would take ten days to two weeks before I would feel the effects. Ten days? Ten more days? He also said that not everyone is helped by Botox. I think he told me that 80 percent of the people injected saw some improvement. Which in my "glass half empty" mind-set meant 20 percent of the people were not helped at all. I began to think, "What if I'm in the 20 percent? What will I do then?" It was not a thrilling revelation.

I remember walking out of the office, still with a booming headache and now with the thirty-five injection points around my head and neck. I was a little disappointed, to say the least. I honestly did not know if I could go another day, let alone ten more days if I was in the 20 percent not helped. Then what would I do? In case you are wondering, at that exact moment I stepped over the line and entered the "far beyond my ability to endure" territory.

The church board leader called me later that week to see how I was doing. He called at a bad moment. I laid it out for him, "I don't know if I can keep going. If Botox is not effective in me, we might have to talk about a leave of absence. I simply cannot keep up in my current condition." We agreed to wait to see what happened (if anything) when the Botox kicked in.

All the while, many people were praying for me. I remember praying, "God, this is it. This is the 'far beyond' point for me. I completely trust you and if Botox doesn't help and if I take a leave of absence, then I will rest in the assurance that you will help me, my family, and the church. I don't see how that could be a good thing. I don't know what I will do. But I am trusting in you."

Those ten days were a nervous, anxious, and painful time.

Then one day I woke up, walked into the bathroom, flipped the light switch, and looked at myself in the mirror.

My face looked different. My forehead was smooth—really smooth. Overnight, the effects of Botox kicked in and there was a lessening of my four-month-old migraine. My headache pain seemed to get a little better each day. The headaches weren't gone, but they were better. The pain was less intense, and there were even days when I didn't have a headache at all. Botox was beginning to break months of a very long headache and bring relief. Praise the Lord!

AT MY LOWEST POINT, GOD ANSWERED MY PRAYER

What if Botox didn't work? What if I was in the 20 percent of headache suffers that do not improve? Then I believe that God would have given me the strength to endure that situation. My ability to make it through those days most certainly would not have come from me—that's for sure. I was already at the "far beyond my ability to endure" point. God obviously knew what I needed, when I needed it, and he came through. He always does.

Maybe you are there right now—the "far beyond your ability to endure" point. If so, then remember the words of Paul to the Romans: "May the God of hope fill you with all joy and peace as you trust in him, so that you may overflow with hope by the power of the Holy Spirit" (Romans 15:13).

I just returned from visiting some missionary friends in Switzerland. It's tough to convince someone that one is "suffering for Jesus" when you are a missionary in Switzerland. It's a gorgeous corner of God's creation. Of course, people living in beautiful countries need Jesus too. So my friends are there.

They live in a little village out in the country, and not far from their house is a dairy farm. What makes this dairy farm special is that there is a machine called a "milk-o-matic" in the barn that is stationed by the road. And for one franc you can place an empty container in the machine and out will come thick, whole, white, yummy milk. It's not straight from the cow, but it's close. If you are a fan of whole milk, then it's the place for you.

While not technically allowed on my diet (and by "not technically" I mean it would not be allowed at all), still I think even my neurologist would have agreed that fresh milk-o-matic ice cold goodness is an unexpected joy. Transforming an empty water bottle into one filled with a yummy, milky bit of heaven is a perfectly good way to break one's diet.

Likewise, God wants to fill you with a bit of heaven. (And it won't cost you a franc, and it doesn't involve a milk-o-matic.) He wants to take your empty, troubled heart and fill it with joy and peace. Heaven is the place when hope turns into reality. The God of hope longs to fill you with overflowing hope while you are on this side of the heavenly shores.

Being filled with an overflowing hope, even while feeling lousy, involves getting your eyes off of the troubles of this world and onto the God of all hope. The one that can fill you to overflowing at the exact moment you need to be filled is ready and able to fill you.

10 | PAIN AND THE PEOPLE YOU MEET
IT TAKES ALL KINDS!

Have you seen the "People of Wal-Mart" email that was circulating a few years back? It purportedly showed individuals shopping at the giant retailer in all manner of clothing and attire that most rational, normal people would not be caught wearing even on Halloween. It confirmed the notion that there are some strange people on planet earth, and at least occasionally, they shop at Wal-Mart.

One can't pastor for nearly twenty-five years (like I have) without having more than a few conversations that left me scratching my head and wondering if aliens did indeed land on Area 51 and are now attending the church I pastor.

People can be irrational, confused, disoriented, and just plain messed up. And most all of them have an opinion about many diverse topics. It may not be an informed opinion. It frequently is not a biblical opinion. But they have opinions.

THE PEOPLE YOU MEET

Unless you are living in a cave as you manage life with chronic pain, you will no doubt cross paths with some people whose attitudes and opinions will contribute to your affliction. If you are part of a family or a faith community or a workplace environment or around people at all, then part of the journey is dealing with such people. Here are just a few of the people that you might encounter along the way. (Disclaimer alert: I refer to each as a "guy," but I use it in a gender-neutral sort of way.)

"Mr. Fix-it" Guy

This person is well meaning and wants his friend to be well. This is an admirable (and only occasionally annoying) quality. So whenever there is a magazine article that deals with your condition; whenever he hears a report on the latest miracle cure; whenever he becomes aware of a news item that has the slightest pain remedy news, this friend passes on the information. (If a friend gave you this book, he is probably a "Mr. Fix-it" guy. Please thank him for me.) These people mean well. If you have a lot of these friends, you will be inundated with remedies and cures. You will know you are loved. Of course, that's a good thing.

Wonderful, loving friends have advised me to eat kale, almonds, peppermint extract, spicy salsa, and watermelon to cure what ails me. Against my doctor's advice, I've been told to drink more caffeine and more orange juice. I've been given homespun concoctions, vitamin supplements, and exercise advice. There has been no shortage of offers for the next great remedy or stories of people who tried some such treatment plan and never again had a headache.

It's good to remember that these people mean well. They are trying to fix your problem. They want to help. They care about their friend. And if the advice is watermelon eating, well, what could it hurt?

"Doubting Worse than Thomas" Guy

This person wonders if you really deal with chronic pain. He might secretly think you are faking it. Pain is an invisible sickness. With pain, there are no scars. No wounds. No visible signs of trouble. "Is your situation really that bad?" he wonders.

Unlike "Mr. Fix-it" guys, these people don't empathize with your plight. They question it. If not outright spoken doubts, in their mannerisms, inquiries, and body language, their questioning attitude is evident.

The best response to "Doubting Worse than Thomas" guy is, "don't sweat it." There is no need to prove or disprove the validity of your ailment. Does it really matter if "Doubting Worse than Thomas" guy fully grasps the pain you endure? Probably not.

"Curious George" Guy

This person loves to ask questions. He isn't malicious or evil—just curious. Where do you hurt? How long does your pain last? Does anything help? How can you sit through a church service with the kind of pain you suffer? They ask questions—lots of questions. HIPAA rules mean nothing to "Curious George" guy.

"Curious George" guy isn't malicious. He can be annoying (depending on how he asks the questions), but generally he is not mean-spirited. The best response to "Curious George" guy is patience and answering the questions you feel comfortable in answering. If the question is a little too personal, simply reply, "That's a little personal." Most people understand. If "Curious George" guy is truly asking the question so that he may better pray for you, then great! The more informed prayers, the better.

Always remember the pain-and-people-interaction life principle: if people want to pray for you, let them! It doesn't matter their denominational preference. If they know Jesus is the healer of humankind, then let them pray. Never say no to someone offering to pray.

"Suspecting Sin" Guy

This person believes verses like Deuteronomy 7:15 ("The LORD will keep you free from every disease") are meant for every person, everywhere, every time. So if you haven't been healed, then the problem obviously can't be God (Hello! God is God), and the only other person involved in the equation is dirty, rotten, stinking you. Hence, you must be the problem. This person reasons, "If God will keep you free from every disease, and if you have a disease (or chronic pain), then you must be the problem."

Much like dealing with "Doubting Worse than Thomas" guy, the pain sufferer doesn't need to get into a theological discussion on how believers could get sick without being sinful. But if biblical examples of those who faithfully suffered various sicknesses are needed, here are a few bullets for your gun. Ask "Suspecting Sin" guy what "sin" Paul committed when he spoke of his "thorn in the flesh." Or what in the world caused Epaphroditus (a guy Paul describes as "my brother, coworker, and fellow soldier") to almost die? When Paul wrote to the Philippians that Epaphroditus was returning to Philippi, he informed the church: "For he longs for all of you and is distressed because you heard he was ill. Indeed he was ill, and almost died" (Philippians 2:26-27). He was a great Christian, but he was sick and nearly died.

In both of these cases, godly, Spirit-filled, fully devoted followers of Christ dealt with sicknesses. You can too. Sickness doesn't equal sinfulness. To think otherwise is not only unwise but also unbiblical.

"Don't Know What to Say" Guy

These people avoid uncomfortable or awkward moments like the plague. They don't know what to say around someone who is suffering. They don't want to say something wrong, so they don't say anything. Often they avoid the sufferer—not because they are unconcerned or uncaring but because they feel very self-conscious about such conversations. They don't want to say the wrong thing (I'm not sure what could be "wrong," but they don't want to say it—whatever it is), so they say nothing.

In dealing with "Don't Know What to Say" guy, disarm the awkward moment by approaching the subject. Let him in on the victories God has given you and offer a few prayer requests. Honesty, Christian love, and humor are the best ways of handling most of these encounters. Remind "Don't Know What to Say" guy that pain is not contagious, but his friendship and conversation is very important to you.

"Head in the Sand" Guy (aka "The Ostrich")

Like "Don't Know What to Say" guy, "Head in the Sand" guy also avoids the sufferer at all costs. Unlike "Don't Know What to Say" guy, he doesn't avoid the pain sufferer because of the awkwardness of the situation; he avoids the pain sufferer because he doesn't want to think about this person. These people act like pain is contagious. Suffering makes them sad. They don't want to be sad, so they would rather ignore the person. "Outta sight, outta mind" is their motto. Self-focused is their perspective.

"Head in the Sand" guy might never be convinced to change. In fact, for these people to totally come around and see the broken and hurting people in his world, God will need to instill in them a compassionate heart. To get their heads out of the sand and into the world, God will need to give them his eyes and his heart.

"Sincere Praying" Guy

As stated before, the best headache interaction life principle is, "If someone wants to pray for you, let him!" This is the one person you want in your life. If someone tells you that he is praying for you and he means it, praise the Lord! If he tells you he is praying every day and he actually does it, then you can have no better friend. If you have a team of people like this in your life, then you are blessed indeed. Gathering many sincerely praying people is an important help in the pain sufferer's life. Get as many folks praying for you as you can get. As I stated earlier, don't ever turn down an opportunity to pray, and don't ever overlook the prayers of a believer when offered.

One of the great blessings in my journey has been the prayer commitment of several friends and people in the church I pastor. They have told me that they pray every day for my health. They constantly have interceded on my behalf. I have no doubts that I managed to travel this migraine mountain as well as I have because of so many people praying for me. It humbles me beyond words to know so many are mentioning me to our heavenly Father. If you can gather such a team, you are blessed indeed!

A BIBLICAL EXAMPLE OF
A SUFFERER AND HIS "FRIENDS"

There was a man in the Bible that had similar "guys" in his life. His problem wasn't pain, but blindness. His story is told in John 9. Here are the *Reader's Digest* facts. A man was born blind. His parents were still living. Because of his condition, he was forced to beg. Jesus saw the man. There is no biblical record of it, but Jesus may have been the first to coin the phrase, "Here's mud in your eye" just before he told the blind guy to put his white cane in a garage sale. (Okay, that last sentence was more imagination than fact, but you get the idea.) Because of his encounter with Jesus, the blind man was blind no more.

In this story, we are also introduced to some of the same type of people I have encountered in my journey. The disciples are the "Curious George" guys. They have questions. Who sinned? Was it this man? (Presumably he had been sinning in the womb since he was born in this condition.) Was it his parents? The accepted theology of the day said sin is the cause of all suffering, so it would have been obvious that someone sinned. The only question for the "Curious George" disciples was "who?"

"Obviously someone displeased God a whole lot for this guy to be born blind. He is a either a dirty, rotten sinner or his folks are dirty, rotten sinners—you don't get this way without somebody being a dirty, rotten sinner, Jesus. So who is it? Who is the awful human being, the man born blind or his folks?"

In all probability, this whole discussion was taking place within earshot of the guy—remember, he was blind, not deaf. And the disciples seemed more concerned about correct theology and philosophical debates than being caring and compassionate toward this man. It's easier to talk about a person than to help the person right in front of them. It's easier to discuss the tragedies of suffering than to help the sufferers.

It happens today—it's easier to complain about the welfare system than to help the poor. It's easier to argue against the evils of abortion than to support an orphanage or care for an unwed mom. It's easier to label than to love. The "Curious George" disciples were guilty of discussing rather than discerning that a man needed Jesus.

The townspeople are the "Head in the Sand" guys. They have distanced themselves so much from this poor man that they can't even agree if the man healed is the same guy they passed by every single day. Which begs the question—who was the real blind beggar? They passed him every single day! Every day they "saw" him, yet they still could not identify him. Ignoring the suffering around them, these people were the picture of the uncompassionate and unconcerned. These townspeople would have won the prize for not being aware of the hurting people in their community.

Again, there are "Head in the Sand" guys in every community and at most every church. Sadly, there are ignored sufferers in every community and at many churches.

Obviously, the Pharisees are the "Suspecting Sin" guys. Only they don't suspect sin—they "know" the former blind guy had sinned. And they believe Jesus sinned. (Making mud pies and healing on Sunday would be exhibit "A" of his "sinful" behavior.) And they suspect his parents were sinners too. "Birds of a feather flock together," they might have said.

What makes this all remarkable is the Pharisees were looking at a guy who was (emphasis on the word *was*) blind—totally blind, blind-from-birth blind. But instead of giving glory to God at the man's healing or instead of rejoicing with the man, they concluded it must be wrong or sinful since the healing didn't fit their methodology.

Have you ever known people like that? They "know" how God works, and any other manner must not be from God. If something doesn't fit into their mold, idea, or methods, then it must be wrong. These are the people who will tell you how to pray for healing and the manner in which to ask for it. They may have charts and methods. In this misunderstanding of healing, those who get well do so because they have followed the right steps with the right words.

This story is a prime example of how Jesus doesn't always work in the same manner. This is the only time he made mud pies to heal a guy. Why did Jesus choose this manner at this time? Who knows? Bottom line—when God heals, it's up to God on the timing, manner, and method in which he does his miraculous work.

The former blind man's parents are the typical "Don't Know What to Say" guys. The former blind guy's parents were brought into the picture. The "Suspecting Sin" Pharisees wanted to know some of the background. They were trying to get to the bottom of this whole healing that "allegedly" took place. "Is this your son? Was he born blind? What's going on here?" It was quite an interrogation.

You get an uneasy feeling that the man's parents in their "Don't Know What to Say" mode did not want to answer too many questions. Yes, he was their son. Yes, he had been born blind. But other than that . . . they weren't talking. They sure weren't willing to go out on a limb for their son, were they? Afraid that they would be booted out of the synagogue, they didn't want to get involved.

It's sad, isn't it? This should have been one of the happiest days of their lives. You can bet they had prayed years and years for this day. "O God, heal our son—let him see! Let our boy know the joy of seeing a sunset or the Milky Way on a starry night. Let him see the waves crashing to shore on the Sea of Galilee, let him see the banners raised on the festival days. Let our boy see!" They had prayed for this type of miracle for years, and on the day when it actually happened, instead of rejoicing, they allow their fears to stifle their joy. How incredibly sad!

It still happens today. There are plenty of people who allow fear, anxieties, and doubts to get the best of them. And in so doing, they are robbed of the joy that could be theirs.

It happens in areas other than asking for healing. Some believers never tell their friends about Jesus for fear of what they would think. So they never experience the joy of seeing a friend accept Christ. When you help someone discover the saving grace of Jesus Christ, it will be one of the greatest days of your life. But it will never happen if fears are robbing you of the opportunity. Others never go on mission trips because they have a weak tummy or are afraid to fly or have one of a million other excuses, but they miss the joy of being a part of what God is doing around the world. And it's sad when believers dealing with excruciating pain (or other debilitating health issues) don't ask to be anointed and prayed over by the community of believers for one of a million reasons (i.e., "I've been prayed over before" or "I don't like to step out from my seat" or "There are other people who are sicker than me"). And the results are predictable—God doesn't answer unprayed prayers.

For the parents of the former blind man, it should have been their happiest day. Instead, their fears got the best of them.

For all we know, the blind guy didn't have a "Sincere Praying" guy in his life, but he still met Jesus, and (understatement alert!) that encounter forever changed his life.

You might have all of these guys in your life (and maybe a few others). I would hope that you would be like the former blind guy in your approach to them.

Do you see his faith journey in John 9? He has moved from thinking of Jesus as a man to referring to Jesus as a prophet in verse 17. A little bit later in verses 30-33 he declares that Jesus is "from God," and finally verse 38 reads: "The man said, 'Lord, I believe,' and he worshiped him."

Because the blind man's parents were so concerned about being "put out of the synagogue" (verse 22), it's probably safe to assume that he was raised in a Jewish home where he was taught there is only one God deserving worship. He no doubt had been taught the Shema from Deuteronomy 6:4-9 that begins: "Hear, O Israel: The Lord our God, the Lord is one." This made his decision to worship Jesus all the more significant. For there was only One deserving of such praise, and the former blind man recognized that he was standing beside him.

I love his response to the Pharisees' declaration that Jesus was a sinner. In verse 25 he basically said, "Listen—you boys are the experts in the theology department. Sinner or not, I don't know. The one thing I do know is I was blind, but now I see. You're the rule keepers. You're the Law experts. What I know is this morning I woke up blind as a bat, but right now I can see the scowl on your face. That's the one thing I know."

What's the one thing you know?

The one thing I know is that without Jesus I'm in trouble. That's what this guy basically said—without him, I'd still be blind. Without him, I'd still be begging. Without him, my life would still be in the dark. "I was blind, but now I see." I'd say the same thing, "Without Jesus my life would be unbearable, but with him even a life with pain can be full, sweet, and blessed."

People may not always understand your plight. They may question, doubt, and have all manner of responses to you. The lesson from the story is to get as close to Jesus as you can possibly get. He is the friend that you can rely upon. He is the one you want in your corner when the pain is raging. He is the one who will not let you down.

11 PAIN AND THE PEOPLE YOU LOVE
YOUR PAIN ISN'T YOURS ALONE

Your pain is not your own. Oh, it is yours all right, but it isn't only yours. Not if you have family and friends. Your pain is theirs too. One person with chronic pain in the family affects the entire family.

When my four-month migraine was raging away, I suffered, but so did my family. I couldn't participate in normal family activities. Frequently I didn't eat with the family. Everyone talked quieter when they were around me. When the TV was on and I was in the room, it was barely audible. Because of the desperation of the situation that summer, I went on the crash migraine diet—but so did my family. They went from Karla's yummy normal dinners to meals with little spices, sauces, or flavor. It was no fun. Not for me. Not for them.

It is natural when in pain to turn your thoughts inward. The natural tendency when suffering is to be consumed with your pain and your issues. It's easy to become self-centered and absorbed in your difficulties. It's imperative to remember—your pain is not yours alone. Other people—the people you love and who love you—are also involved in your pain. It wreaks havoc with your loved ones too.

Jesus' suffering on the cross not only speaks of God's salvation plan for the world but also gives a great example of how to be selfless in the midst of pain. Of the seven words from the cross, three deal with relationships with the people near him. (I will deal with the other four comments from the cross in chapter 12.) Jesus gave a great example of how we can be involved and respond to the people in our lives when dealing with troubles and sufferings (including pain).

READY TO FORGIVE

When gazing upon those people who put him on the cross and who were mocking his very existence, Jesus said, "Father, forgive them, for they do not know what they are doing" (Luke 23:34). There was no anger, malice, or revenge in his heart. There was no animosity or resentment.

When in pain it is easy to want to find someone or something to blame. It is easy to become bitter with life. The natural reaction is to be angry when others don't understand your plight or have little regard for your well-being. But such feelings and attitudes only increase our suffering.

I remember just after my brain hemorrhage I was lying in the intensive care unit of the hospital. The room was dark. Every pin drop was like a cannon going off in my head. At that moment out in the hallway, no doubt unaware of my situation or my proximity to their conversation, two hospital workers were having a wonderfully exuberant conversation. They were laughing and carrying on. Under normal circumstances, I probably would have wanted to join in. I don't remember what their conversation was about, but I don't recall it as being anything but a normal conversation between friends.

The longer the conversation continued, the more frustrated I became. "Don't they know this is a hospital? Isn't there a 'Quiet Please' sign somewhere? How can they not know that people with brain injuries (it was a brain injury ICU) cannot tolerate noises?"

Somewhere in the middle of the conversation that lasted probably ten minutes (but at the time it seemed like an hour to me) it dawned on me how unproductive my frustrations were. I was unable to get up from the bed. I could not speak loud enough from my bed to interrupt their conversation and let them know I was unhappy with their volume. Any attempt I might have made would have caused more pain than what I was already experiencing. To grow increasingly angry over a matter that was not evil or intentional or even wrong was a little silly. I decided my best option was to put the pillow over my head and wait. To not sweat the noise and trust that it would end soon. It did, and I felt much better just for letting the frustration go.

Forgiving people or giving them the benefit of the doubt puts our heart at ease. Trying to keep straight who wronged you, why they wronged you, and how you will get back at them for wronging you is a pain in itself. Let it go. Forgive where forgiveness is needed and cut some slack where that is needed.

Don't blame—bless.

Don't find fault—offer grace.

Don't dole out your own version of pain—give mercy.

Jesus had plenty of reason to not forgive the mob surrounding him, but he did forgive in the midst of suffering. We would do well to do the same.

READY TO ENCOURAGE

The second statement from the cross in the midst of Jesus' suffering went to the man nearest to him—to one of the thieves. Following the thief's question about Jesus remembering him in paradise, Jesus said (in so many words, "I'll do better than remember you"), "Truly I tell you, today you will be with me in paradise" (Luke 23:43).

Was there a more hopeless person on the planet at that moment than this thief? By his own admission, he was guilty. Whatever he was accused of doing, he did it. He said, "We are punished justly, for we are getting what our deeds deserve" (Luke 23:41). As such, he had a few hours (at most) to live.

Again, Jesus could have been thinking of his own imminent death. He could have been consumed with the pain and suffering he was enduring. He could have been in deep thought on the big picture and the salvation of humankind. He would have many reasons not to be concerned for a convicted, guilty thug. But in his suffering, far from turning self-centered in his own dilemma, Jesus offered hope to a hopeless man.

There are always people near you that need an encouraging word, a prayer prayed on their behalf, or a willing and generous heart able to meet a need. When we get our eyes off our own suffering and see the needs around us and when we set our course on making a difference and being a help to others, that is when our suffering becomes less of a burden.

One memorable migraine took place on a night we had planned to go to a rescue mission to serve dinners to the homeless men of Kansas City. I debated whether I should go. My head was pounding, and the mission would be filled with hungry and loud men. Maybe I should pass this time around. Our church sends a crew each month; I would have plenty of opportunities to serve.

I decided to go. This is another time when I didn't want the migraine to win. I did not want to lose this battle. Throughout the drive (about thirty minutes) I was wondering if I had made the right decision. Once at the mission, my tasks included chopping vegetables, setting the tables, and making the place ready for the men that would soon arrive for dinner. The headache did not subside. Quite to the contrary, the smells from the kitchen and the mission were making me more and more nauseous. I remember praying a quick prayer, "Lord, I'm here to serve. Help me to serve."

As the men started to arrive, I was taking them their trays of food. I would try to strike up conversation and smile a lot. It was busy that night. There were a lot of trays to be delivered and a lot of small talk being offered. Somewhere in the serving and the talking, I realized my head was not raging like it was twenty minutes earlier. It still hurt, but the nausea and noise of the dining area was no longer consuming.

Maybe the medications I had taken were finally kicking in. Or maybe, just maybe, when I got my attention off my light and momentary troubles and on to those men who were hungry and needed a bed to sleep in that night, the pain decreased. When consumed with ourselves, our pain seems greater. When serving and thinking of others, our headaches or other ailments become less than consuming.

Here's what I eventually came to believe. My migraine was going to be with me whether or not I was kind and courteous. So why not be kind and courteous? If I refuse to allow the headache to win and instead serve others (again, I understand some pain renders us incapable of doing anything), God will honor that service.

You don't have to find a rescue mission to discover this truth. There are people to serve all around you: to the pharmacist that is giving you your medication, be encouraging and thank him or her for helping in your struggle. To the mail carrier, offer a cool drink in the summer or a warm drink in the winter. To your family members and friends, determine to not neglect their situations and frustrations. If you are going to have a headache anyway, then do your best (with God's strength) to be positive, encouraging, helpful, and kind.

READY TO RESPOND

The third saying of Jesus from the cross has the strongest implications for dealing with the people we love during our times of struggle and suffering. It was the words Jesus said to his mother, Mary, and John, his beloved disciple. "Dear woman, here is your son. . . . Here is your mother" (John 19:26-27, NLT). Even while dying on the cross, Jesus did not forget his responsibilities to his mother. In our life struggles we can do the same.

My Aunt Alice was a great example of a person who had every reason to focus on her sufferings but instead thought of her family and their well-being. Her example and the result of her faithfulness in the midst of her suffering was nothing short of amazing.

I guess everybody has a favorite relative. Mine was Aunt Alice. She always gave the best birthday and Christmas presents. When other relatives gave dopey shirts or underwear, Aunt Alice always seemed to know what I wanted. Her birthday cards always had a little bit more money in them than the other birthday cards. Her refrigerator was always stocked with Faygo pop (for you non-Michiganders, Faygo was a tasty Detroit brand of soda; my favorite was Faygo Root Beer and my brother's favorite was Faygo Rock and Rye), and she and my uncle had a swimming pool (which was very nice for the two weeks of mildly warm weather we had each summer in Michigan).

Growing up, we went to her house (which was always immaculately clean) on most Friday nights and nearly every Sunday afternoon. Occasionally, we'd stay over on Sunday afternoons and go to church with her at night. She always had peppermint Life Savers in her purse that helped keep me quiet in church. Every Christmas, the Prince family gathering was at her house. We would crowd around a shiny silver metallic Christmas tree with revolving color lights and open presents and eat food and laugh and laugh. I have nothing but fond memories of my aunt and being at her house every weekend.

My admiration for my aunt goes far beyond presents, swimming pools, or Faygo soda. Looking back now, I realize that my Aunt Alice did not have an easy life. She grew up during the depression with alcoholic parents. There was little money and when her mother died (the result of her alcoholism), Alice, though still a child, assumed the role of homemaker and mother to her two brothers. My Uncle Jim, her younger brother, was an epileptic and had frequent grand mal seizures. He contracted polio that left him crippled, and after a brain injury he had the mental capacity of a small child. It could not have been an easy task to be his primary caregiver, but my aunt did it. In her late teenage years, she got married to her teenage sweetheart and, knowing the homelife that she was leaving, she invited her brother (my dad) to live with her and her brand-new husband. How many newlyweds would want an eight-year-old kid hanging around? My dad moved in with them, but during his teen years, he started following the example of his father before him and dropped out of high school, joined a gang, and became an alcoholic. I'm sure he was the cause of much anxiety and sleepless nights for my aunt.

My Aunt Alice's worries were not limited to her siblings and an alcoholic father. With two young children at home and my dad a rebellious teenager, World War II began, and her husband was drafted into the army and quickly shipped overseas to fight the Nazis. One day, a telegram arrived telling her that my Uncle Dick was killed in action. Two or three weeks later, she received another telegram saying the army had made a mistake—my uncle was not dead but had been captured by the Germans and was a prisoner of war. Imagine the two terrible weeks of thinking you are a widow with two small children to raise, followed by months of worry about the torture and hardships that your husband was forced to endure. When my uncle was finally liberated by the Americans at the end of WW II, he weighed less than a hundred pounds. He returned to the States and soon afterward, my aunt became pregnant. Life seemed to be improving. But the baby she was carrying died soon after birth, and one week later, her twelve-year-old daughter also died of rheumatic fever.

I've tried to put myself in her shoes. How would I handle the seemingly never-ending battles, heartaches, worries, and grief? There were no medications to help relieve the stress, no counselors she could call upon, not even Oprah or Dr. Phil and their homespun gobbledygook on TV. Amazingly, she was never defined by her struggles. The hardships she endured and the difficulties she faced didn't make her bitter or harden her heart. In fact, she took those trials as opportunities to rely upon the Lord even more, and in so doing she not only overcame the trials of her life but became even more compassionate and more concerned about others.

My aunt was a wonderful Christian lady who had a sweet, joyful spirit. For as long as I could remember, she was her little church's treasurer. She looked on this role as a sacred duty to handle the Lord's money as a good steward. Even when the passing of years and ill health made it so she could no longer attend services, every week she would write out her tithe check and make sure it got put into the offering plate at her church.

As I look on her life and faith, I realize she is the one who changed the entire course of a family. She is the one who broke the generational pull of alcoholism and started a new course for generations to follow. The statistics say most often the children of alcoholics will follow in those footsteps. But she did not.

She became a Christ follower when a boy invited her to a Sunday school picnic. That boy, my Uncle Dick, later became her husband. I don't know if the potato salad was any good, but she found Jesus and a husband! That was some picnic! The generations that have followed have continued to follow Christ in her footsteps. My father, because of a sister who prayed and wouldn't give up on him (she was an Epaphras-type of prayer warrior), became a Christ follower and was redeemed and rescued from alcoholism. My brother and sisters are all serving the Lord. (My brother and I are both pastors.) Our children are all serving the Lord.

All of my aunt's children are also serving the Lord. Her oldest son accepted the Lord soon before his death a few years ago, and so her prayers were answered for all of her children's salvation. One son is a pastor and two of her grandchildren are also serving as pastors.

My entire family can trace our Christian roots back to this woman of incredible faith who refused to allow the horrible things of life to define her; rather, she chose to look to Christ as her hope and help. She refused to become self-absorbed by her own struggles but was determined to be a shining light. Any one of the burdens in her life could have caused her to become bitter and angry, but instead she was a blessing to her family, her church, and anyone she encountered.

That's how I want to be as I struggle with chronic pain. I don't want pain to define me and my relationships. My family would tell you that sometimes I go overboard when I am battling a migraine. I try so hard for it to not overtake me— for it not to win. I try to convince myself that if I don't give in, the headache will go away. That strategy rarely works. But there have been plenty of times when, through God's help, I have not allowed a headache to defeat me, and I have been able to participate in and enjoy family times.

Chronic pain may be a part of your life; you may know all too well times of suffering; and if so, then learn from Jesus on the cross as he approached the people in his life. He was quick to forgive, encouraged others, and responded in love, grace, and truth. In the next chapter, we will look at the four other words from the cross and see from them how Jesus in his suffering offered encouragement for the unique challenges of pastoring a church while navigating the paths with chronic pain.

12 | PAIN AND THE MINISTER
BEING A SPIRITUAL LEADER WHILE IN PAIN

Being a pastor has its share of headaches even if one is not prone to migraines. I will freely admit that I am thankful that my headaches are the result of a brain hemorrhage, food triggers, the weather, and genetics but are rarely the result of (okay, occasionally they are helped along by) unruly church members, uncertain finances, or trouble at home—in other words, things that won't always be remedied by Botox and other medications.

PAIN AND THE WORSHIP WARS

Pastoring with pain presents unique challenges for the minister. For example, in the church I pastor we have three distinctly different worship services: a somewhat-traditional, a somewhat-contemporary, and a somewhat-rock-and-roll type of service. Should a parishioner with a pounding headache not attend the somewhat traditional service because our organist loves to open up the stops and let the organ boom every now and then, that is his or her choice. Or should the parishioner decide to not attend the rock-and-roll service because of the volume—well, he or she has other options. But the pastor with a booming headache just has to grin and bear it. (Please understand I love all three of our services but occasionally each one has contributed to a migraine.) Pain does not have a favorite in the worship wars in many of our churches. It is equally annoyed with all styles. Maybe a Quaker service of quietness would be the best worship style for the pain-prone minister. But of course, we can't all be Quakers.

I've never quite figured out what triggers my migraines, but it seems that they frequently strike at inopportune times. Sometimes they come with little warning or regard to the importance of the particular moment. My two most memorable massive headaches during a worship service occurred on a Christmas Eve service and a Mother's Day Sunday. Calling in sick wasn't an option on either of those days. So what do you do? I took some medication, grinned, prayed, and trusted that the Lord would get me through the service without my saying anything too weird in my medicated state. Of course, the Lord did help—by helping I mean I made it through the services and I don't think too many people were aware of what was raging in my melon.

PAIN AND THE PASTORAL REALITIES

Pain issues for the pastor are not limited to the drums and the organ in worship services. The daily duties of pastoring when struggling with chronic pain can be draining and at times close to debilitating. More than the pain and physical issues, there are plenty of emotional and spiritual issues that can hinder the pain-suffering pastor's ability to effectively minister.

Once again, Jesus' words from the cross give great insight for the pastor who is suffering from pain (or any other issue, for that matter). I have already addressed three of his words in the previous chapter—the other four statements from the cross can be a tremendous help to the suffering pastor.

WHEN FEELING ALONE

Pastoring can be one of the loneliest professions even in the best of times. In the worst of times and in the times of suffering, it can be excruciatingly lonely. That's why it is good for the pastor to hear the words from the cross. In Matthew 27:46 Jesus said, "My God, my God, why have you forsaken me?"

Given my light sensitivity and need to be in a dimly lit room when a headache is raging, it has been good for me to remember that Jesus spoke these words when the world was covered in total darkness. Isolated and suffering, Jesus cried out from the darkness to God. He knows deep loneliness and the feelings of being abandoned. He asked the mammoth question of all who have ever suffered, "Why, God? Why have you forsaken me?" In other words, when feeling the most alone, the most isolated, the most misunderstood, know this: Jesus understands. He's been there.

It wasn't only Jesus who suffered from times of great loneliness in the Bible. David, Jeremiah, and the apostle Paul all wrote about their struggle with loneliness. Jeremiah sums up how I have felt when the migraine seemed to be winning:

> I wish my head were a well of water
>> and my eyes fountains of tears
> So I could weep day and night
>> for casualties among my dear, dear people.
> At times I wish I had a wilderness hut,
>> a backwoods cabin,
> Where I could get away from my people
>> and never see them again. (Jeremiah 9:1-2, TM)

Why bring up this point? If you struggle with loneliness and feelings of isolation—if those feelings are exacerbated by pain, you are not alone. Loneliness comes. Not because of sin. Paul, Timothy, and Epaphroditus all battled sickness without sin. Jesus, David, Jeremiah, and Paul were exactly where God would have them at that point in their lives and yet they had times of loneliness. Loneliness does not equal sinfulness.

So what does that tell you?

It should tell you that just as your pain might not be the result of sin, neither is the corresponding loneliness that can accompany it.

If some of the greatest, godliest people that ever walked on the planet dealt with loneliness (and of course, if Jesus himself could cry out from a lonely state), then you and I can be lonely too.

Loneliness is not always the result of something we did or did not do; sometimes loneliness just happens. Sometimes it is the result of the suffering we are enduring. But the quicker we can acknowledge it, the more we are able to move on to God's way of dealing with it.

The notion of thirty to forty sharp needles piercing one's noggin like I receive in the Botox injections actually sounds worse than it is. It sounds like I am a human pincushion—and I guess I am. But it's really not that bad. Take that from a guy who absolutely hates needles. But my way of dealing with thirty to forty shots to the head and neck in one sitting at the doctor's office is to close my eyes as tight as possible and pretend that I am not getting thirty to forty shots in my head.

As soon as the doctor comes in, I jump on the examining table, close my eyes tight, and keep them shut. I have had several series of treatments, and I have yet to see a needle. In my little mind game, I think if I don't see it, if I close my eyes really, really tightly, and if I can make small talk with the doctor and his assistant, then maybe the injections are not happening.

That approach works for me in the forty-five minutes I am in the neurologist's office, but that is not the best approach to take with loneliness: pretending it's not there, refusing to acknowledge the loneliness, and thinking it will go away is a bad method for finding relief.

It's a bad method because it just doesn't work.

Just as refusing to look at the needles doesn't make them go away (I don't look but I still feel each and every injection), refusing to acknowledge our loneliness doesn't make the pain go away. It's still there. Unlike my Botox injections, where the pain of the shots is temporary and the relief it brings is so worth it, loneliness pain is often not temporary and it brings absolutely no relief.

Instead of pretending that we are not lonely, we need to learn from God's Word and hold on tight to God's promises. David, a man after God's own heart and a man who knew a thing or two about loneliness, modeled what we are to do in Psalm 25. He said:

My eyes are ever on the LORD,
for only he will release my feet from the snare.
Turn to me and be gracious to me,
for I am lonely and afflicted.
Relieve the troubles of my heart
and free me from my anguish. (Verses 15-17)

When the pain is raging and you are feeling like you are alone and no one understands your plight, turn your eyes to the Lord. He's been there. He knows your lonely heart's cry, and he can do something about it.

WHEN TEMPTED TO THINK YOU HAVE TO BE SUPERMAN (OR SUPERWOMAN)

One of the myths that many pastors believe is that they have to be Superman. Oh, maybe not the whole cape-and-tights-wearing thing, but they function as if they are required to have Superman-like qualities. As if the old TV show began with these words:

She is stronger than a carnal board member;
Faster than a speeding toddler escaping from the nursery;
Able to leap tall pews in single bound.
She's Superpastor!

I hate to be the one to break this to you. You are not Superpastor. And when you are in constant pain, you are really not Superpastor. But that's okay. God hasn't called you to be Superpastor. He has called you to pastor with all of your frailties and limitations.

Jesus' next statement from the cross reminds us of this point—while suffering and dying on the cross, Jesus simply said in John 19:28, "I am thirsty." In those three words, he showed he was not exempt from the limitations and troubles of this world. There is no avoiding pain while living on this earth. It is part of what it means to be human. While dying on the cross, Jesus (fully divine and fully man) experienced the very real need of thirst. He wasn't a superhero. He wasn't above needing the basic things of life.

When a headache is raging (a dark room, no sound, sick-to-my-stomach type of migraine), I feel pretty helpless. At that moment I know I am not Superpastor and that I need help. I don't like to admit it, but it helps to negate any feelings of resentfulness or feeling of being a burden to know that Jesus as he was suffering asked for a drink.

There is no shame in asking for help. There is no shame in being vulnerable, honest, and admitting that you are not Superpastor. You are a real person with real issues and real struggles. There are times when humbling oneself and asking for help is a great example in dealing with suffering for the rest of the believers in your congregation. Others in your church suffer too. Often they suffer in silence. As the pastor models openness, honesty, and vulnerability, walls can be broken down in the congregation.

I have been very open with my headache issues. (It's kind of hard to hide a brain hemorrhage, I know.) But I've been open with the continuing struggle. HIPAA laws have been thrown out the window. I share with my congregation (when appropriate) not to muster up feelings of sorrow or woe, but to remind the people that none of us have everything together. All of us have issues. Mine are headaches. Theirs may be something else. Bottom line—we all are in need of a Savior.

Part of the pain relief is allowing people to be a blessing to you. Ask for help when it's needed. Receive the help when offered. You are not Superpastor. You were not called to be a Superpastor. So don't act like you are Superpastor.

WHEN WONDERING ABOUT THE PURPOSE OF IT ALL

The constant struggle with pain can lead very quickly to a defeatist place. Will this pain ever end? What good could possibly be the result of my struggle? Is God hearing my pleas? Doesn't God know that if I were 100 percent healthy, I could accomplish many more things for him?

Jesus reminds us in his three-word proclamation from the cross in John 19:30 that our struggles are not in vain. He said, "It is finished." His mission was accomplished. He did what the Father had planned.

Our suffering is not in vain either. It, too, can accomplish what the Father has in mind. As the pastor continues to live on full of grace and truth in spite of the pain, God will produce his desired outcome.

Am I a better pastor because of my headaches? That's a question I have asked myself many times. I've concluded I am. I am more understanding of those that struggle with pain. I am more empathetic to the burdens and issues of suffering. I am more aware of the hopelessness that can grip even believers' hearts when there is a daily, constant attack against them. I've stated earlier I pray more these days and am in the Word more. Of all the measures that I can think of, I am better because of the pain. Again, that's not to say I want it. I would eliminate it faster than Usain Bolt can grab a gold medal. Still, I see where God has used my plight to help others. Mission accomplished!

WHEN LONGING FOR AN END

No doubt, as the pain continues, the natural, inevitable question becomes, "How long will I endure this?" As we discussed in the chapter about the calendar, I don't have an answer to that question. But here's what Jesus reminds us from the cross. It's not forever. His last word from the cross is found in Luke 23:46: "Father, into your hands I commit my spirit."

Pain is not forever, and death does not have the final word. Jesus died in the exact same place as he lived—squarely in the Father's hands. Every pastor knows that not every prayer uttered for healing results in healing in this life. What we can be assured of is that all pastors struggling with pain or any other issue when living their lives to please and honor God can rest knowing, whether or not healed, they are in the hands of God.

Pastoring with pain requires patience, endurance, and a whole lot of God's grace. I find strength in my calling that I received as a young teenager. I know God called me to do what I am doing. When I sensed God's calling, I was sitting by a campfire at a church campground. That moment is as clear in my mind thirty-five years later as it was then. I know God has called me to do what I am doing.

Furthermore, when God called me he knew about that defective blood vessel in my brain that would one day burst. He knew all about the headaches, medications, and Botox. He knew all of my defects and issues. But he still called me. And if you are pastoring with pain, I would encourage you to hold on to the calling that God has placed upon you. Remind God of that moment in your life, and call upon him to give you the strength and grace you need for every day.

God called you, pastor. You are not doing what you do because of a whim or a wish. Pastoring is a calling. God called you—pain and all. Because this is true, God will give you the grace and strength for this moment to accomplish his purpose and goals through you.

13 | PAIN AND HOPE
KEEP ON BELIEVING

The question I've been repeatedly asked by those who are aware of my migraine troubles is: How can you do it? How can you keep on going? How can you keep smiling, working, and ministering? Obviously, if you have been reading this book, then you know it is not me but Christ in me. No question. No doubt. I am able to press on solely because of Jesus empowering and enabling me. The most important attribute that he continues to instill in me is hope.

Whatever a migraine may throw at me, the old song is still true: "My hope is based on nothing less than Jesus' blood and righteousness."

In Romans 8, Paul is writing to a group of people living in the capital city of the pagan Roman government. When Paul wrote this letter, Nero was the emperor. In a few years, he would burn the city of Rome and blame the Christians for its destruction. It wasn't an easy place to live and be a Christian.

Tradition says that both Peter and Paul were executed in Rome—obviously Rome was not an easy place to be a follower of Jesus. The culture and society were less than welcoming to their teaching and worldview.

No doubt as Paul was writing to these believers, they were already being persecuted. They were already the subject of prejudice and contempt. So Paul wrote to this group of believers and said:

What, then, shall we say in response to these things? If God is for us, who can be against us? He who did not spare his own Son, but gave him up for us all—how will he not also, along with him, graciously give us all things? Who will bring any charge against those whom God has chosen? It is God who justifies. Who then is the one who condemns? No one. Christ Jesus who died—more than that, who was raised to life—is at the right hand of God and is also interceding for us. Who shall separate us from the love of Christ? Shall trouble or hardship or persecution or famine or nakedness or danger or sword? As it is written:

"For your sake we face death all day long;
we are considered as sheep to be slaughtered."

No, in all these things we are more than conquerors through him who loved us. For I am convinced that neither death nor life, neither angels nor demons, neither the present nor the future, nor any powers, neither height nor depth, nor anything else in all creation, will be able to separate us from the love of God that is in Christ Jesus our Lord. (Romans 8:31-39)

Don't you love this passage? "If God is for us, who can be against us?" And when God is for us, "we are more than conquerors"! That's what Paul said. Read it and rejoice: "we are more than conquerors"!

We are not described as sufferers.

We are not just survivors.

We are not just those who are hanging on until the sweet by and by.

We are victors: "More than conquerors." What does that mean? Isn't it enough to just be a conqueror? Why does Paul say we are "more than conquerors"?

To conquer means you have won.

To conquer means you have dominated.

To be a conqueror means you haven't just won a battle; you've completely won the war! Have a ticker tape parade. It's party time. The fighting is over.

But to be more than a conqueror means not only have you won but you have taken over. You have enjoyed all the spoils of the war. To be more than a conqueror means you have achieved all that there is to achieve and then some. That's what being more than a conqueror means.

And Paul is saying, if God is for you (and he is for you), then who in the world can be against you? If God is for you (and he is for you), then even the scariest things this old world can fling at you—trouble or hardship or persecution or famine or nakedness or danger or even the sword—will not have the final word! I think you can include pain on that list. Maybe chronic pain sufferers should read that verse this way: "Who shall separate us from the love of Christ? Shall trouble or aches or dizziness or nausea or loud noises?" No! We are more than conquerors!

God is for us. He is not against us. Pain rages. God is still for us. Migraine is blasting away, but he has not forgotten us. You say, "I don't feel like a 'more than conqueror.'" You are!

Believer—be strong! Be excited. Be invigorated! God is for us! One hundred percent for us!

This morning was my day for a run. In a matter of full disclosure, the doctors have been encouraging me to exercise for years, but I didn't take the advice seriously until the last several months. Now I run a couple of miles three or four days a week. I don't really like running. I don't see where it helps my head all that much, but it does help my heart, and now I am in better shape than I was several months ago. So now I run.

I had two big problems as I was beginning my run. The first problem was that last night I had a massive headache. Really bad. Usually when I have such a headache, the next morning I have a hangover. I am glad to say that my hangovers have never been the result of something I drank the night before. So problem number one was the "morning after" residual head troubles pounding around in my head.

Why run with a headache, you ask? That was my excuse when the doctors kept encouraging me to exercise. I kept thinking, "I don't want to run with a headache—I want to be in bed with the covers pulled over my head, not outside pounding the pavement." So I never ran. Then it dawned on me—if I only exercised if I did not have a headache, I would rarely exercise (maybe once or twice a week). You can't establish healthy patterns if you are only doing it once a week. So I determined headache or no headache, I was going to run. And since I have started, I can only recall one time when I physically could not run at all because of a migraine. I have cut short runs several times because of headaches, but as stated previously I had decided that headaches would not win in this exercise battle. So, hangover headache raging, I decided to run anyway.

The second problem was that when I got outside to run, it was misting just a little bit. I know that there are head cases (no pun intended) that like to run in the rain. I am not one of them. But the mist was so light, I wasn't even sure if it was really misting. The ground was dry. "Maybe it's not really misting," I convinced myself. It was cloudy, but it did not appear that rain was imminent. So I ran.

I got about a mile and a half into my planned three-mile run when the weather changed from a "misting—maybe, maybe not" kind of rain, not quite to a "raining cats and dogs, Noah and the flood" kind of rain, but a steady, "you are nuts to be running in the rain" kind of rain. I was halfway into my run, which meant I had another fifteen minutes of running. (Real runners please note: I acknowledge that if one is "running" a ten-minute mile pace it might not be considered "running.") Running or not, it was not going to be a pleasant fifteen minutes.

My options were limited. There was no Starbucks I could run into to wait out the storm (thereby disproving the theory that there is a Starbucks on every corner). There were no big floppy trees I could wait under. My options were: run in the rain or wait in the rain. I decided to run. With each step I was thinking, "Just keep going. You are one step closer to home. Don't stop. Keep running. Don't think about the weather. Just keep running."

I am sure that more than one of the drivers in the cars that passed me as I was running thought, "Look at that goofball running in the rain. He must be one of those head cases that likes running in the rain." None stopped to see if I would rather be dry in their car with a ride home. So I ran on. Finally, soggy and sore, I made it home. (In another manner of full disclosure, I do not normally run three miles. Usually I run two miles, but I wanted to go a little farther that day because I was preparing for my first 5K race.)

You may feel similar to me when it started to rain at this point in your life journey. Pain or troubles have left you feeling like you are exhausted, uncomfortable, and a long way from home. My advice to you is what I told myself in the rain: "Just keep going. You are one step closer to home. Don't stop."

Like my running in the rain, there might not be a great option available to you. There might not be a place where you can rest from your journey and troubles. There might not even be a little stop-off place that leaves you mostly high and dry. Just keep going. With each step you are one step closer to home. God is with you on each and every step of your journey. So keep going.

The author of Hebrews put it this way: "Let us run with endurance the race God has set before us. We do this by keeping our eyes on Jesus, the champion who initiates and perfects our faith" (Hebrews 12:1-2, NLT). He didn't say run with ease or run with no pain, but run with endurance. To endure means that there are struggles that you are enduring. So keep running the race. If God has chosen not to instantly and miraculously heal you, then run the course that he has set out before you. You will make it. A good day is coming. The finish line is near. Just keep running!

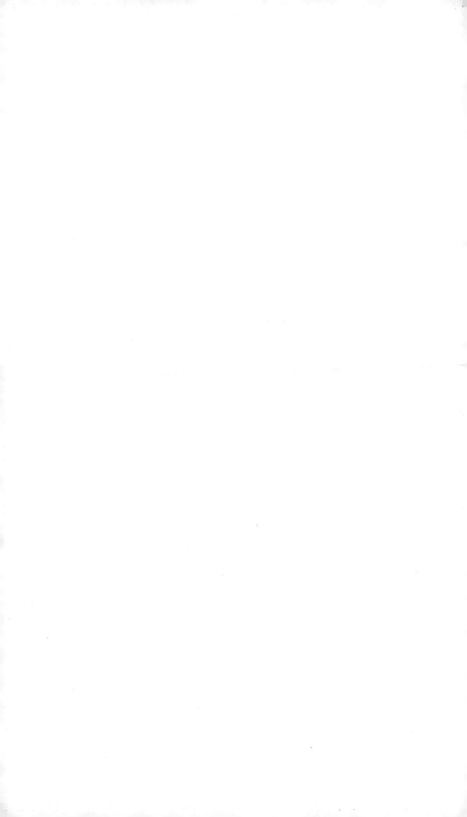